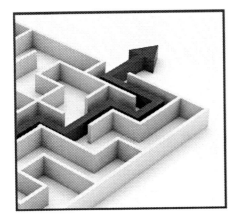

MW01247786

Environm Tracer Workbook

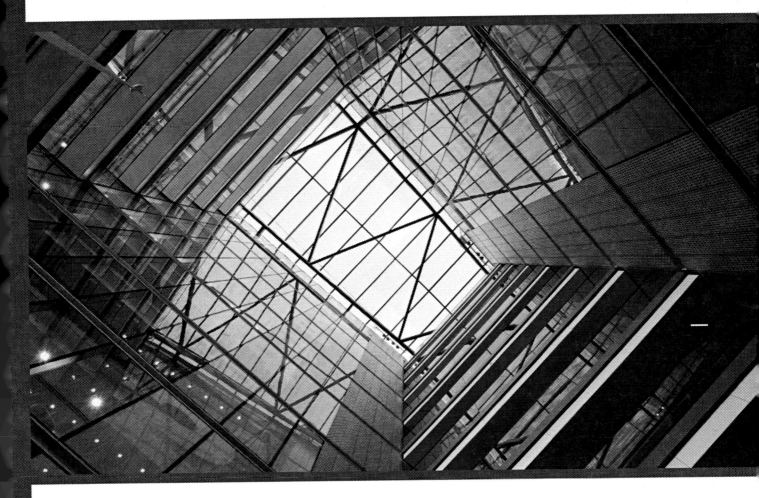

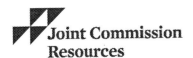
Joint Commission
Resources

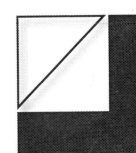

Executive Editor: Kristine M. Miller, M.F.A.
Project Manager: Bridget Chambers
Manager, Publications: Lisa Abel
Associate Director, Production: Johanna Harris
Executive Director: Catherine Chopp Hinckley, Ph.D.

Joint Commission Reviewers: George Mills, M.B.A., F.A.S.H.E., C.E.M., C.H.F.M., Senior Engineer, Standards Interpretation Group; Jerry Gervais, C.H.F.M., C.H.S.P., Associate Director/Engineer, Standards Interpretation Group; John Fishbeck, R.A., Associate Director, Division of Standards and Survey Methods; Lynne Bergero, M.H.S.A., Project Director, Department of Standards and Survey Methods; Jerry Dykman, Surveyor, HAS; Stephen Turner, C.H.S.P., *Life Safety Code* Specialist, Accreditation and Certification Operations

Joint Commission Resources Reviewer: Lisa Abel, Manager, Publications

---

Joint Commission Resources Mission

The mission of Joint Commission Resources is to continuously improve the safety and quality of care in the United States and in the international community through the provision of education and consultation services and international accreditation.

Joint Commission Resources educational programs and publications support, but are separate from, the accreditation activities of The Joint Commission. Attendees at Joint Commission Resources educational programs and purchasers of Joint Commission Resources publications receive no special consideration or treatment in, or confidential information about, the accreditation process.

The inclusion of an organization name, a product, or a service in a Joint Commission publication should not be construed as an endorsement of such organization, product, or service, nor is failure to include an organization name, a product, or a service to be construed as disapproval.

This publication is designed to provide accurate and authoritative information regarding the subject matter covered. Every attempt has been made to ensure accuracy at the time of publication; however, please note that laws, regulations, and standards are subject to change. Please also note that some of the examples in this publication are specific to the laws and regulations of the locality of the facility. The information and examples in this publication are provided with the understanding that the publisher is not engaged in providing medical, legal, or other professional advice. If any such assistance is desired, the services of a competent professional person should be sought.

ISBN: 978-1-59940-611-4

Library of Congress Control Number: 2011925859

For more information about Joint Commission Resources, please visit http://www.jcrinc.com.

Table of Contents

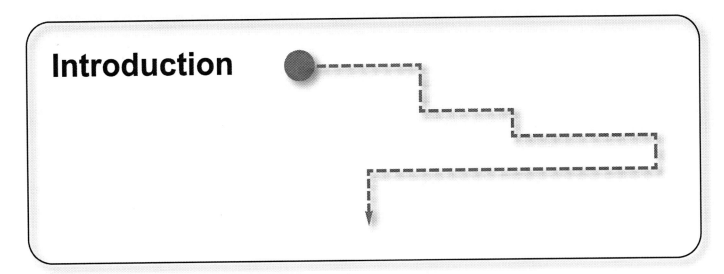

Introduction

Tracer methodology is an integral part of the on-site accreditation survey process used by The Joint Commission and Joint Commission International (JCI). Surveyors use tracers to evaluate the care of an individual or to evaluate a specific care process as part of a larger system. A surveyor reviews an individual's record and follows the specific care processes the individual experienced by observing and talking with staff members in areas where the individual received care. This methodology provides the surveyor with an opportunity to assess the organization's systems for providing care and services and its compliance with accreditation requirements. This book, part of a series that focuses on familiarizing health care staff with tracer methodology, can help an organization learn to conduct simulated—or mock—tracers that mimic actual tracers. The mock tracer is conducted by someone in the organization who performs the role of an actual surveyor.

Benefits of Understanding Tracers

Health care organizations that educate staff about tracers will have a better understanding of the overall survey process, especially since an on-site surveyor can typically devote up to 60% of his or her time conducting tracers. In addition, an organization that understands tracers can use mock tracers as a tool to assess its compliance with standards and make improvements before a surveyor arrives. For example, if an organization wants to analyze how well a specific aspect of a system on a specific unit functions—such as the security in the neonatal intensive care unit of a hospital—it can conduct a mock tracer of that system. Although its purpose would be to learn more about how systems function in that particular unit, a mock tracer

would also provide important information that could identify broader issues for improvement.

Types of Tracers

Surveyors currently conduct three types of tracers:

- *Individual:* An individual tracer follows the actual experience of an individual who received care, treatment, or services in a health care organization (that is, a patient, a resident, or an individual served). To select individuals to trace in U.S. health care organizations, surveyors take into account an organization's clinical/service groups (CSGs) and its top priority focus areas (PFAs) identified through the Joint Commission's Priority Focus Process. The CSGs categorize care recipients and selected services into distinct populations for which data can be collected. PFAs are processes, systems, or structures in a health care organization that significantly impact safety and/or the quality of care provided (*see* Appendix A). The organization's specific CSGs and PFAs inform the choice of what types of areas, units, services, departments, programs, or homes to visit initially to conduct an individual tracer; the CSGs, in turn, help the surveyor select an individual to trace. Although information from the Priority Focus Process may help surveyors select the first individuals and areas to trace, a surveyor may trace the experience of additional care recipients based on the initial findings during the on-site survey.

- *System based:* A surveyor may use a system-based tracer to analyze a high-risk process or system across an entire organization to evaluate how and how well that system functions. Currently, there are three topics explored during the on-site survey using the system tracer approach: medication management, infection control, and data management. To analyze a medication management or infection control system, a surveyor can follow an individual's actual care experience through the organization and assess how well that particular system functioned related to that individual's care. But to analyze a data management system, the surveyor conducts a group meeting session and focuses on assessing an organization's use of data in improving safety and quality of care. The goal of a data management system tracer is to learn about an organization's performance improvement process, including the organization, control, and use of data. There is no individual care recipient to follow; however, data from performance improvement are used and evaluated during the course of individual tracers throughout a survey.

- *Program specific:* A surveyor may use a program-specific tracer to analyze the unique characteristics and relevant issues of a specific type of organization. The goal of this type of tracer is to identify safety concerns in different levels and types of care. For example, a patient flow tracer is a program-specific tracer used in hospitals, whereas a continuity of care tracer is a program-specific tracer used in an ambulatory care organization.

A survey may also include an **environment of care (EC) tracer.** Like a system tracer, this type of tracer examines organizational systems and processes—in this case, systems related to the physical environment. This book focuses on EC tracers.

Second Generation Tracers

During any type of tracer, a surveyor may see something involving a high-risk area that requires a more in-depth look. At that point, the surveyor may decide to conduct a second generation tracer, which is a deep and detailed exploration of a particular area, process, or subject. These types of tracers are a natural evolution of the existing tracer process.

The following are high-risk topics in hospitals and critical access hospitals that surveyors might explore in more detail using a second generation tracer approach: cleaning, disinfection, and sterilization (CDS); patient flow across care continuum; contracted services; diagnostic imaging; and ongoing professional practice evaluation (OPPE)/focused professional practice evaluation (FPPE).

Tracers Used Internationally

Tracer methodology is being used to assess health care organizations beyond the United States. Health care organizations that undergo JCI accreditation also experience tracer methodology when surveyors visit their facilities. The concept is essentially the same for both domestic and international organizations; however, there are slight differences. Whereas U.S. surveyors use such elements as PFAs and CSGs to select care recipients to trace, these criteria do not apply to international surveys. JCI surveyors use information provided in the organization's accreditation survey application to select tracer subjects from an active care recipient list. Subjects typically selected are those who have received multiple or complex services because they, most likely, have had more contact with various departments of the organization, providing a greater opportunity for the surveyor to assess how systems work in the organization. Furthermore, program-specific tracers are done as part of "undetermined survey activity" appropriate to an organization, as defined in the *JCI Survey Process Guide.* Also, international organizations refer to the EC tracers as "facility management and safety" tracers and to data management system tracers as "improvement in quality and patient safety" tracers.

Conducting Mock Tracers

The best way to understand all types of tracers is through practice—that is, through conducting mock tracers. This involves developing some basic skills, such as learning how to ask good questions. An actual tracer is not performed by one person in isolation. It involves talking with multiple staff members and, in the case of individual tracers and some system tracers, the care recipient and even family members (if possible) to learn details about an individual's health care experience or how a particular system functions in an organization. All important details about the individual's care or the system's function can be explored by asking simple questions in succession. And how a question is asked is particularly important. A surveyor poses questions in a manner that encourages the staff member or care recipient to share as much information as possible. Observation of the surroundings or attention to how a respondent answers one question can lead to other related issues and can trigger additional questions.

Skills in analysis and organization are also involved, particularly in planning a mock tracer, and of course, analysis is necessary to evaluate and prioritize the results of a mock tracer. Similar skills are involved in the reporting of the results and in the follow-up on any consequent plans for improvement based on the results. Often, an organization will institute a mock tracer program that will train participants for optimum outcomes to these practice tracers. The benefits that result from mock tracers support and enhance the continuation of such teams.

How to Use This Book

We designed the *Environment of Care® Tracer Workbook* to help staff members in all health care settings better understand how EC tracers work and how to conduct mock tracers:

- "How to Conduct a Mock Tracer" follows this Introduction. It provides step-by-step instruction on performing a mock tracer.

- The Overview that follows "How to Conduct a Mock Tracer" goes into further detail about EC tracers.

- Each section of this workbook includes examples of tracers, called *scenarios*, that address specific EC, emergency management (EM), or life safety (LS) topics.

- Each scenario is preceded by a list of the PFAs that emerge during the scenario. Then, a narrative describes how a surveyor might analyze the particular EC system.

- Sample tracer questions follow each scenario. They show the types of questions a surveyor might ask staff members or other individuals for the specific scenario. These questions are keyed to the narrative to show how and when they might occur during the scenario.

- Each section also includes an example of a tracer worksheet that utilizes the sample tracer questions from one scenario and shows how the worksheet might be completed during mock tracer activities.

- Each scenario includes helpful sidebars that provide compliance and mock tracer tips.

- Appendixes describe the PFAs and provide forms that are helpful in developing a mock tracer program.

Acknowledgments

A work of this scope requires a concerted team effort. This book, which we hope you find to be as useful as it is practical, could not have been created without such a team. We are indebted to our writer, Kathleen B. Vega, for her attention to detail and her outstanding professionalism.

We are also grateful to our Joint Commission reviewers (*see* page ii) for their thorough and timely input.

How to Conduct a Mock Tracer

The main activity during a Joint Commission or Joint Commission International (JCI) survey of any type of health care organization is the tracer (*see* the sidebar "Tracers at a Glance," at right). A **mock tracer** is a practice tracer meant to simulate an actual tracer. During a mock tracer, one or more people may play the role of a surveyor. Some organizations develop teams of such "surveyors" and repeatedly conduct mock tracers as part of an ongoing mock tracer program.

Mock tracers are done for several reasons:
- To evaluate the effectiveness of an organization's policies and procedures
- To engage staff in looking for opportunities to improve processes
- To be certain the organization has addressed compliance issues and is ready for survey at any time

What follows is a 10-step primer for how to conduct a mock tracer. It addresses the process in four phases:
- Planning and preparing for the mock tracer
- Conducting and evaluating the mock tracer
- Analyzing and reporting the results of the mock tracer
- Applying the results of the mock tracer

Each step within these phases includes suggested approaches and activities. You might want to use the "Mock Tracer Checklist and Time Line" on page 7 to guide you through the phases. The primer also explains how to use the scenarios, sample worksheets, and appendixes in this workbook to conduct mock tracers. Note that the primer can be modified to suit any health care organization.

Tracers at a Glance

Duration: A Joint Commission individual tracer (*see* "Individual Tracer" on page 6) is scheduled to take 60 to 90 minutes but may take several hours. During a typical 3-day survey, a surveyor or survey team may complete several tracers; during a single-day survey, it may be possible to complete only one or two tracers. Tracers constitute about 60% of the survey.

Survey team: A typical Joint Commission survey team includes one or more surveyors with expertise in the organization's accreditation program. For domestic (not international) hospitals and critical access hospitals, a *Life Safety Code*®* Specialist is also part of the team. A team leader is assigned for any survey with more than one surveyor. A surveyor typically conducts a tracer on his or her own and later meets up with the rest of the team to discuss findings.

Tracer activity: During tracer activity, surveyors evaluate the following:
- Compliance with Joint Commission standards and National Patient Safety Goals and, **JCI** for international organizations, JCI standards and International Patient Safety Goals
- Consistent adherence to organization policy and consistent implementation of procedures
- Communication within and between departments/ programs/services
- Staff competency for assignments and workload capacity

(continued)

* Life Safety Code *is a registered trademark of the National Fire Protection Association, Quincy, MA.*

Tracers at a Glance (continued)

- The physical environment as it relates to the safety of care recipients, visitors, and staff

Range of observation: During a tracer, the surveyor(s) may visit (and revisit) any department/program/service or area of the organization related to the care of the individual served or to the functioning of a system.

Individual tracers: Individual (patient) tracer activity usually includes observing care, treatment, or services and associated processes; reviewing open or closed medical records related to the care recipient's care, treatment, or services and other processes, as well as examining other documents; and interviewing staff as well as care recipients and their families. An individual tracer follows (traces) one care recipient throughout his or her care in the organization.

System tracers: A system tracer relates to a high-risk system or the processes that make up that system in an organization. Currently, three topics are explored during the on-site survey using the system tracer approach: medication management, infection control, and data management. The data management system tracer is the only tracer that is routinely scheduled to occur on regular surveys for most organizations; it may include evaluation of data for medication management and infection control, as well. Other system tracers take place based on the duration of the on-site survey; the type of care, treatment, or services provided by the organization; and the organization's accreditation history. Lab accreditation programs do not have system tracers. **JCI** In international organizations, data system tracers are called "improvement in quality and patient safety" tracers and are not individual based.

Program-specific tracers: These are tracers that focus on topics pertinent to a particular accreditation program and the associated care, treatment, or service processes. These processes are explored through the experience of a care recipient who has needed or may have a future need for the organization's care, treatment, or services. Examples include patient flow in a hospital or suicide

prevention at a residential program. Lab accreditation programs do not have program-specific tracers.

Environment of care tracers: Although the environment of care (EC) tracer is not one of the defined Joint Commission system tracers, it is similar to those types of tracers. Like system tracers, EC tracers examine organization systems and processes—in this case, systems related to the physical environment, emergency management, and life safety. Also, like system tracers, an EC tracer is often triggered by something observed during an individual tracer, as surveyors notice environmental-, emergency management–, and life safety–based risks associated with a care recipient and the staff providing care, treatment, or services to that person. A surveyor may also be assigned to do an EC tracer as part of a comprehensive survey process. Note that EC tracers are performed only in facility-based accreditation programs and do not apply to community-based programs and services, such as those provided by some behavioral health care accreditation programs. **JCI** For international organizations, EC is referred to as "facility management and safety."

Second generation tracers: A surveyor may see something during a tracer involving select high-risk areas that requires a more in-depth look. At that point, the surveyor may decide to conduct a second generation tracer, which is a deep and detailed exploration of a particular area, process, or subject.

Planning and Preparing for the Mock Tracer

Step 1: Establish a Schedule for the Mock Tracer

Careful planning is necessary for any successful activity, including a mock tracer. Consider the following when establishing a schedule for mock tracers in your organization:

- *Schedule by phase:* Allow adequate time for each phase of a mock tracer. The focus of each phase outlined in this primer is shown in the checklist "Mock Tracer Checklist and Time Line" (see page 7) with suggested time frames, some of which may overlap. Suggested approaches and activities for each phase comprise the remainder of this primer.

Mock Tracer Checklist and Timeline

✔	Planning and Preparing for the Mock Tracer	
	Step 1: Establish a Schedule for the Mock Tracer	Month 1
	Step 2: Determine the Scope of the Mock Tracer	Month 1
	Step 3: Choose Those Playing the Roles of Surveyors	Month 1
	Step 4: Train Those Playing the Roles of Surveyors	Month 1 and 2
✔	**Conducting and Evaluating the Mock Tracer**	
	Step 5: Assign the Mock Tracer	Month 2
	Step 6: Conduct the Mock Tracer	Month 3
	Step 7: Debrief About the Mock Tracer Process	Month 3
✔	**Analyzing and Reporting the Results of the Mock Tracer**	
	Step 8: Organize and Analyze the Results of the Mock Tracer	Month 4
	Step 9: Report the Results of the Mock Tracer	Month 4
✔	**Applying the Results of the Mock Tracer**	
	Step 10: Develop and Implement Improvement Plans	Months 5–7

Note: *To follow up on findings and sustain the gains, periodically repeat mock tracers on the same subjects.*

- *Make it part of your regular PI program:* Make mock tracers part of your ongoing performance improvement (PI) program. Schedule mock tracers for different departments/ programs/services several times a year.

- *Share the plan with everyone:* Let everyone in your organization know about the mock tracers being planned. No set dates need to be given if the mock tracers are to be unannounced, but communication about planned and ongoing mock tracers is necessary for recruitment of those who will play the roles of surveyors and for cooperation from all departments/programs/services.

- *Understand the Joint Commission survey agenda:* A mock tracer typically simulates only the tracer portion of a survey, which constitutes the foundation of the survey. By understanding the survey activities, however, those who are

playing the roles of surveyors can better simulate tracers to help your organization prepare for a survey. Joint Commission surveys follow a tight agenda. Check the *Survey Activity Guide* (SAG) for your accreditation program(s). The guide outlines what happens in each survey activity. All accreditation program SAGs are posted on the Web site for The Joint Commission. They are also available on your *Joint Commission Connect*™ extranet site if yours is an accredited health care organization or an organization seeking Joint Commission accreditation. **JCI** International organizations should consult the *International Survey Process Guide* (SPG), which is sent to applicants seeking international accreditation and is also available to order on the JCI Web site.

- *Relate it to the date of the last survey:* Joint Commission surveys are typically conducted on a regular, triennial basis. For most accredited organizations, the survey will occur within 18 to 36 months after an organization's last survey, although laboratory surveys and certification program reviews are on a two-year cycle. With the exception of critical access hospitals and office-based surgery practices, organizations accredited by The Joint Commission must conduct Periodic Performance Reviews (PPRs) between full surveys. The PPR is a management tool that helps the organization incorporate Joint Commission standards as part of routine operations and ongoing quality improvement efforts, supporting a continuous accreditation process. A mock tracer can help by giving the organization more insight into compliance issues. Conducting the mock tracer before a survey date allows time to address compliance issues prior to the PPR deadline; conducting a mock tracer shortly after the last survey is helpful for assessing compliance with problems highlighted in that recent survey. Note that the PPR is not applicable to the Medicare/Medicaid certification–based long term care accreditation program. **JCI** For international organizations, the survey will occur within 45 days before or after the accreditation expiration date. International certification programs are on a three-year review cycle. Also, although international organizations are not required to complete PPRs, JCI recommends that organizations do a self-assessment of compliance between surveys. (International certification programs have a required intra-cycle review process.)

Step 2: Determine the Scope of the Mock Tracer

Assess your organization to determine where to focus attention. By listing problems and issues in your organization, the scope of the mock tracer—whether comprehensive or limited—will become clear. One or more of the following approaches may be used to determine a mock tracer's scope:

- *Imitate the Priority Focus Process:* The Priority Focus Process (PFP) provides a summary of the top clinical/service groups (CSGs) and priority focus areas (PFAs) for an organization. The CSGs categorize care recipients and/or services into distinct populations for which data can be collected. The PFAs are processes, systems, or structures in a health care organization that significantly impact safety and/or the quality of care provided (*see* Appendix A). The PFP is accessible on the *Joint Commission Connect* site for domestic organizations and provides organizations with the same information that surveyors have when they conduct on-site evaluations. Address all or some of the areas generated in that report. **JCI** International organizations do not have PFPs; however, it may be helpful and important to look at your last survey results and target areas of greatest concern.

- *Reflect your organization:* Start with your organization's mission, scope of care, range of treatment or services, and population(s) served. Choose representative tracers that support and define your organization.

- *Target the top compliance issues:* Review the Joint Commission's top 10 standards compliance issues, published regularly in *The Joint Commission Perspectives®* (available for subscription and provided free to all accredited organizations). Also check any issues highlighted in *Sentinel Events Alerts,* which are available on the Joint Commission Web site, at http://www.jointcommission.org/sentinel_events.aspx. Address compliance issues that are also problem prone in your organization. Be especially mindful to note if any of these top compliance issues have been noted in current or past PPRs. **JCI** International organizations can request top compliance issues from this address: JCIAccreditation@jcrinc.com.

- *Review what is new:* Address any new Joint Commission or JCI standards that relate to your organization. New standards and requirements are highlighted in the binder version (although not in the spiral-bound book version) of the most recent update of the *Comprehensive Accreditation Manual* for your program. Also focus on any new equipment or new programs or services in your organization. Consider mock tracers that will allow opportunities to evaluate newly implemented or controversial or problematic organization policies and procedures and how consistently they are being followed.

- *Start with the subject:* Look at typical tracers from any past surveys and choose several common or relevant examples for the types of tracers defined in the Introduction to this workbook. Or, if your organization has never had a survey, consider the guidelines described in the sidebar "Choosing Tracer Subjects" on pages 9–10.

- *Cover the highs and lows:* Focus on high-volume/high-risk and low-volume/high-risk areas and activities. Ask questions about demographics for those areas or activities to help determine whether care, treatment, or services are targeted to a particular age group or diagnostic/condition category. Then pick corresponding tracer subjects.

- *Target time-sensitive tasks:* Look at time-sensitive tasks, such frequency of staff performance evaluations, critical result reporting, and the signing, dating, and timing of physician orders, including whether they are present and complete. These are often challenging compliance areas.

• *Examine vulnerable population(s):* Review the risks in serving particularly vulnerable, fragile, or unstable populations in your organization. Select tracer subjects (care recipients, systems, or processes) that might reveal possible failing outcomes. Address related processes of care, treatment, or services that are investigational, new, or otherwise especially risky.

Step 3: Choose Those Playing the Roles of Surveyors

If your goal is to conduct more than one mock tracer, either concurrently or sequentially, you will want to develop a mock tracer team. Careful selection of those playing the roles of surveyors is critical. A general guide for a mock tracer team is to follow the number and configuration of your last Joint Commission or JCI survey team (*see* the sidebar "Tracers at a Glance" on page 5). However, you might want to involve more people or have multiple mock tracer teams; try to allow as many people as possible to be exposed to the tracer process and to learn more about the surveyors' angle on the process. If your organization has not had a survey yet, aim for five to eight team members, or select one team member for each department/program/service in your organization plus one for each type of system tracer and one for the EC. Consider the following when choosing those who will play the roles of surveyors:

• *Include administrators:* Administrators, managers, and other leadership should be not only supportive of mock tracers but also involved. Include at least one administrator or manager on the team. Include executive-level leaders in the early stages to provide input and model team leadership. Also, staff may need time off from their regular duties to participate in various phases of a mock tracer, so team members should be sure to get the approval of their managers.

• *Select quality-focused communicators:* Sharp, focused professionals with excellent communication skills are needed to play the roles of surveyors. Recruit people who are observant, detail oriented, and committed to quality and professionalism. Those playing the roles of surveyors should be articulate, polite, personable, and able to write clearly and succinctly. They should be comfortable talking to frontline staff, administrators, and care recipients and families.

• *Draw from committees:* Often the best choices for those who will play the roles of surveyors have already been identified and serve on various committees in your organization. Draw from committee members to find top-notch candidates.

• *Don't forget physicians:* Because they are a critical part of any health care organization, physicians should be involved

---

Choosing Tracer Subjects

Individual tracers: For individual mock tracers, adopt the way actual surveyors choose care recipients. In U.S. health care organizations, select them based on criteria such as (1) whether they are from the top CSGs in the PFP; (2) whether their experience of care, treatment, or services allows the surveyor to access as many areas of the organization as possible; (3) whether they qualify under the criteria for any accreditation program–specific tracer topic areas; or (4) whether they move between and receive care, treatment, or services in multiple programs, sites, or levels of care within your organization. Also, consider tracing care recipients who have been recently admitted or who are due for discharge. **JCI** In international organizations, use information provided in your organization's accreditation survey application to select tracer care recipients from an active list that shows who has received multiple or complex services.

System tracers: Care recipients selected for tracing a system typically reflect those who present opportunities to explore both the routine processes and potential challenges to the system. For example, to evaluate medication management systems, select care recipients who have complex medication regimens, who are receiving high-risk medications, or who have had an adverse drug reaction. To evaluate infection control, select someone who is isolated or who is under contact precautions due to an existing infection or compromised immunity. These same care recipients could be the subjects for data management system tracers, as each might be included in performance measurement activities such as infection control surveillance or adverse drug-reaction monitoring data. **JCI** In international organizations, data system tracers are called "improvement in quality and patient safety" tracers and are not individual based.

Program-specific tracers: The focus for these tracers may include programs such as foster care, patient flow, continuity of care, fall reduction, and

(continued)

Choosing Tracer Subjects (continued)

suicide prevention. For example, to evaluate a fall-reduction program in a long term care facility, you would select a resident identified as being at risk for falls to trace components of the program, such as care recipient education, risk assessment, and falls data.

Environment of care tracers: Subjects for an EC mock tracer may include systems and processes for safety, security, hazardous materials and waste, fire safety, utilities, and medical equipment. For example, an EC mock tracer might examine the security in the neonatal intensive care unit, the safety of hazardous materials that enter through the loading dock, or the installation of and maintenance for new medical equipment. Be sure also to include emergency management life safety issues as topics for mock tracers. **JCI** In international organizations, EC is referred to as "facility management and safety."

Second generation tracers: Subjects for second generation tracers grow naturally out of tracers involving high-risk areas because this type of tracer is a deeper and more detailed exploration of the tracer subject. Areas subject to second generation tracers include cleaning, disinfection, and sterilization (CDS); patient flow across care continuum; contracted services; diagnostic imaging; and ongoing professional practice evaluation (OPPE)/focused professional practice evaluation (FPPE).

in mock tracers—and not always just as interview subjects. Recruit physicians to perform the roles of surveyors. This angle of participation will not only allow them to *apply* their expertise and experience but will also allow them to *add* to that expertise and experience.

- *Draft from HR, IM, and other departments or services:* Those playing the roles of surveyors may also be drafted from among the staff and managers of nonclinical departments, including human resources (HR) and information management (IM). Housekeeping and maintenance staff are often valuable as "surveyors" for their unique perspective of daily operations.

Step 4: Train Those Playing the Roles of Surveyors

All staff trained to portray surveyors need to have both an overview and more detailed knowledge of tracers as part of their training. Even those who have been through a survey need training to play the role of a surveyor. Those who will be acting as surveyors should do the following as part of their training:

- *Get an overview:* Take some time to learn the basics of tracers. The Introduction to this workbook provides a good overview. As a next step, read the *Survey Activity Guide* for your program, which is posted on the Web site for The Joint Commission and on *Joint Commission Connect*. The guide explains what surveyors do in each part of the different types of tracers. **JCI** The JCI *Survey Process Guides* are provided to international organizations applying for accreditation and are also for sale on the JCI Web site.

- *Learn the standards:* Challenging as it may be, it is essential that those who are playing surveyors become familiar with current Joint Commission requirements related to the targeted tracer. They must gain a solid understanding of the related standards, National Patient Safety Goals, and Accreditation Participation Requirements. To learn about changes and updates to Joint Commission standards and how to interpret and apply them, they should read the monthly newsletter *Joint Commission Perspectives* (available for subscription and provided free to all domestic accredited organizations). Be particularly careful to give those who are playing surveyors sufficient time to learn the standards for the department or area in which they will conduct a mock tracer. At least one month is advised (*see* the sidebar "Mock Tracer Checklist and Time Line" on page 7). **JCI** International organizations should be familiar with JCI standards and International Patient Safety Goals, as outlined in the current relevant JCI accreditation manual. Updates, tips, and more are provided free via the online periodical *JCI Insight*.

- *Welcome experience:* Staff and leaders who have been through a tracer can be valuable resources. Invite them to speak to the tracer team about their experiences with tracers and with surveys in general.

- *Examine closed medical records:* Closed medical records are an excellent practice tool for individual tracers and individual-based system tracers. Examine closed (but recent) records and then brainstorm the types of observations, document review, and questions that a surveyor might use to trace the subject of the record.

- *Study mock tracer scenarios:* Tracer scenarios, like those in this workbook, will help familiarize team members with the general flow of a tracer as well as the specific and unique nature of most tracers. The questions that follow each tracer scenario in this workbook can be used to populate a form for a mock tracer on a similar subject in your organization (*see* Appendix B). The sample tracer worksheet at the end of each section in this workbook provides a model for how someone playing the role of a surveyor might complete a worksheet based on such questions. **JCI** Issues addressed in scenarios for domestic settings may be transferable to international settings.

- *Practice interviewing:* Since a large part of a tracer is spent in conversation, people who are filling the roles of surveyors should practice interviewing each other. Although these people should already be good communicators, a review of common interview techniques may be helpful (*see* the sidebar "Interviewing Techniques" at the right).

Conducting and Evaluating the Mock Tracer

Step 5: Assign the Mock Tracer

A mock tracer team may have one member play the roles of surveyor in a specific mock tracer, or the team members may take turns playing the role during the tracer. With repeated mock tracers, every team member should have the opportunity to play a surveyor. Consider these options when assigning role-playing surveyors to mock tracers:

- *Match the expert to the subject:* Match a "surveyor" who is an expert in a department/program/service to a mock tracer for a similar department/program/service—but for objectivity, do not assign them to the same specific department/program/service in which they work.

- *Mismatch the expert to the subject:* Match a "surveyor" to a department/program/service that is new to him or her. This may enhance the objective perspective. Of course, that person will have to prepare in advance to become familiar with the requirements for that new department/program/service.

- *Pair up or monitor:* Pair "surveyors" so they can learn from and support each other, or allow one "surveyor" to follow and monitor the other for additional experience. One of those in the pair might be the mock tracer team leader.

Interviewing Techniques

- Take your time. Speak slowly and carefully.
- To help set the interview subject at ease, try mirroring: Adjust your volume, tone, and pace to match those of the person to whom you are speaking. (If the subject is nervous or defensive, however, use a quiet and calm approach to encourage that person to match your example.)
- Use "I" statements ("I think," "I see") to avoid appearing to challenge or blame the interview subject.
- Ask open-ended questions (to avoid "yes/no" answers).
- Pause before responding to a subject's answer to wait for more information.
- Listen attentively, nodding to show you understand.
- Listen actively, restating the subject's words as necessary for clarification.
- Manage your reactions to difficult situations and avoid using a confrontational tone, even if your subject sets such a tone. Take a deep breath and wait at least three seconds before responding.
- Always thank your interview subject for his or her time and information.

Step 6: Conduct the Mock Tracer

All departments/programs/services in your organization should already have been notified about the possibility of staff conducting mock tracers. Unless mock tracers are announced, however, there is no need to notify interview subjects when the tracer is scheduled to occur. During the mock tracer, team members should do the following:

- *Collect data:* Like real surveyors, those playing the roles of surveyors must collect data that help to establish whether your organization is in compliance with applicable accreditation requirements. They should do this by taking notes on their observations, conversations, and review of documents. Notes may be entered on an electronic form (using a laptop computer) or on a paper form.

- *Be methodical and detail oriented:* To help establish and simulate an actual tracer, those portraying surveyors should strive to be as methodical and detail oriented as actual surveyors. The following techniques may be useful:

○ Map a route through the mock tracer, showing who will be interviewed in each area. It is helpful to interview the person who actually performed the function targeted by the tracer, but any person who performs the same function can be interviewed.

○ Identify who will be interviewed in each area, using specific names (if staffing schedules are available) or general staff titles. For example, if you have singled out a particular care recipient to trace, identify which staff members cared for that care recipient. Of course, this may not be possible to do because staff to be interviewed may depend on what is found in the targeted area, where the care recipient travels within the organization, and what procedures are performed.

○ Note the approximate amount of time to be spent in each department/program/service. That will help keep the tracer on schedule. Notwithstanding any tentative scheduling of the tracer, however, you may uncover unexpected findings that will necessitate either spending more time in a particular location or going to locations that were unforeseen at the time the tracer started. Flexibility is a key attribute of a good surveyor doing tracers.

○ Take notes on a form, worksheet, or chart developed by the team for the purpose of the mock tracer. (The mock tracer worksheet form in Appendix B can be used for this purpose.)

○ Surveyors are directed to be observant about EC issues. Some EC issues may be photographed for the record, provided that no care recipients are included in the photos.

• *Share the purpose:* Whenever possible, remind tracer interview subjects of the purpose of tracers and mock tracers: to learn how well a process or system is functioning (not to punish a particular staff member or department/program/ service).

• *Maintain focus:* Keep the process on track and continually make connections to the broader issues affecting care recipient safety and delivery of care, treatment, or services.

• *Be flexible and productive:* If a person playing the role of a surveyor arrives in an area and has to wait for a particular interview subject, that time can be filled productively by interviewing other staff and making relevant observations and notes. If more than one mock tracer is scheduled for the same

day—as in a real survey—"surveyors" may cross paths in an area. One "surveyor" should leave and return at a later time.

• *Address tracer problems:* Be prepared to identify and address any problems with the mock tracer process encountered during the mock tracer, including practical arrangements (such as the logistics of finding appropriate staff), department/program/service cooperation, team dynamics, and staying on schedule. Decide in advance whether to address such problems in an ad hoc fashion (as they are encountered) or as part of a debriefing after the mock tracer to prepare for subsequent mock tracers.

Step 7: Debrief About the Mock Tracer Process

After each mock tracer, and particularly after the first few, meet as a team as soon as possible to evaluate and document how it went. (Note: This debriefing session should focus on the mock tracer process, not what the mock tracer revealed about your organization's problems or issues. That will be done in Step 8: "Organize and Analyze the Results of the Mock Tracer"; *see* below.) You may choose to use one of the following approaches:

• *Hold an open forum:* An open forum should allow all team members to discuss anything about the tracer, such as methods, logistics, and conflict resolution. For a broader perspective, invite interview subjects from the mock tracer to participate.

• *Let each member present:* In a direct, focused approach, team members can present their feedback to the rest of the team, one at a time. Each person playing the role of a surveyor can be given a set amount of time to present, with questions to follow at the end of each presentation.

• *Fill out a feedback form:* Team members and mock tracer participants can complete a feedback form in which they record their impressions of the mock tracer and suggestions for improvement of the process. These can be vetted and then discussed at the next team meeting to plan for the next mock tracer.

Analyzing and Reporting the Results of the Mock Tracer

Step 8: Organize and Analyze the Results of the Mock Tracer

Conducting a mock tracer is not enough; the information gained from it must be organized and analyzed. The problems and issues revealed in the mock tracer must be reviewed, ranked, and prioritized. You might want to use one or more of the following suggested methods to do this:

- *File the forms:* If the mock tracer team used forms—either electronic or paper (such as the form in Appendix B), those can be categorized for review. The forms might be categorized by types of problems/issues or by department/program/service.

- *Preview the data:* Those who played the roles of surveyors should be the first to review the data (notes) they collected during the mock tracer. They should check for and correct errors in the recording of information and highlight what they consider to be issues of special concern.

- *Rank and prioritize the problems:* The team, led by the team leader, must carefully evaluate all of the team's data. Critical issues or trends can be identified and then ranked by severity/urgency with regard to threats to life or safety, standards noncompliance, and violations of other policies. Prioritizing is the next step and will require considerations such as the following:
  o What is the threat to health or safety? What is the degree of threat posed by the problem—immediate, possible, or remote?

  o What is the compliance level? Is the problem completely out of compliance? That is, does the problem relate to a standard that always requires full compliance (that is, Category A standards) or one for which you may be scored partially compliant or insufficiently compliant (that is, Category C standards)?

  o What resources are required? How much staff time and resources will likely be needed to correct the problem? Depending on the threat to health or safety and compliance level, there may be a time limit imposed on how soon the problem must be corrected (for example, immediately or within 45 or 60 days).

Step 9: Report the Results of the Mock Tracer

An organization's reaction to a mock tracer will depend largely on the results of the mock tracer, including how—and how well—the results are reported. In all reports, it is important to avoid having the tracer appear punitive or like an inspection, so do not include staff names or other identifying information. Following are several ways to report results effectively:

- *Publish a formal report:* Compile all documents and carefully edit them. Determine which documents most clearly summarize the issues. Submit a copy of the report to the appropriate leadership.

- *Present as a panel:* Invite leadership to a panel presentation in which team members present the results of the tracer—by department/program/service or by other arrangement (for example, problems with staffing, infection control, handoff communication, or transitions in care, treatment, or services).

- *Call a conference:* Set up an internal conference event in which you present the results. They could be presented on paper, delivered by speakers from a podium, and/or delivered using audiovisual formats. Invite leadership and everyone who participated in the mock tracer. Keep the conference brief (no more than two hours), being considerate of attendees' time. Make the content easier to digest by color-coding the level of priority and using other keys to signal the types of problems and their severity. Open up the conference to feedback with breakout brainstorming sessions on how to address the problems.

- *Post for feedback:* Post the results on a secure organization intranet and ask for feedback and suggestions from participants and others in your organization. A bulletin board in the lunchroom works, too. After a week, remove the report and incorporate any new information to present to leadership.

- *Report in a timely way:* One goal of a mock tracer is survey preparedness via standards compliance, so addressing problems before a survey is vital. All reports should therefore be made within one month after completion of a mock tracer to allow plenty of time to correct compliance problems.

- *Accentuate the positive:* Remember to pass on positive feedback that comes to light during the mock tracer and data analysis. To encourage continued success as well as future positive interactions with the mock tracer process, reward or acknowledge departments and individuals that participate or are especially cooperative and responsive.

Applying the Results of the Mock Tracer

Step 10: Develop and Implement Improvement Plans

Your reports should indicate which problems must be addressed immediately and which can wait, which require minimal effort to correct and which require extensive effort. Employ one or more of the following improvement plan approaches to help address corrective actions:

- *Hand off to managers:* Hand off any easily addressed corrective actions that are particular to one department/ program/service to the relevant managers. Inform them of your estimates of time and resources necessary to address the problem. Offer to work with them on more complex corrective actions. Offer to repeat mock tracers to confirm findings.

- *Work with PI:* Most of what will need to be done will require integration into your organization's PI program. Follow the required approach in addressing corrective actions.

- *Check your compliance measures:* Be sure to check which elements of performance (EPs) for a Joint Commission standard require a Measure of Success (MOS). These are marked with an **Ⓜ**. At least one measure demonstrating the effectiveness of recommended changes should be included in the action plans addressing compliance for those EPs with an **Ⓜ**, and it must be included if the findings will be integrated into a PPR. **JCI** There is no MOS for JCI standards. Standards are Fully Met, Partially Met, Not Met, or Not Applicable. JCI requests that a Strategic Improvement Plan (SIP) be developed by the organization for any Not Met standard(s)/measurable element(s) and/or International Patient Safety Goal(s) cited in the survey report when the organization meets the conditions for accreditation. In-

ternational organizations do not complete PPRs. (*See* the discussion of PPRs in "Relate It to the Date of the Last Survey," under "Step 1: Establish a Schedule for the Mock Tracer," on page 8.)

- *Share the plans:* Make sure the entire organization is aware of the corrective actions proposed as a result of the mock tracer. Cooperation and support during future mock tracers depend on awareness of their value and follow-through. Activities and results can be shared in internal newsletters or staff meetings.

- *Monitor the plans:* The mock tracer team is not responsible for completing all the corrective actions, but it is responsible for working toward that goal by monitoring any plans based on findings from the mock tracer. Give deadlines to heads of departments/programs/services and others involved in corrective actions (in accordance with any PI policies). Check regularly on progress and make reports to leadership and the PI program on progress and cooperation.

- *Prepare for the next round:* After a few mock tracers, most organizations discover the exponential value of such exercises. They then develop a mock tracer program that allows for periodic mock tracers, sometimes with several running at one time.

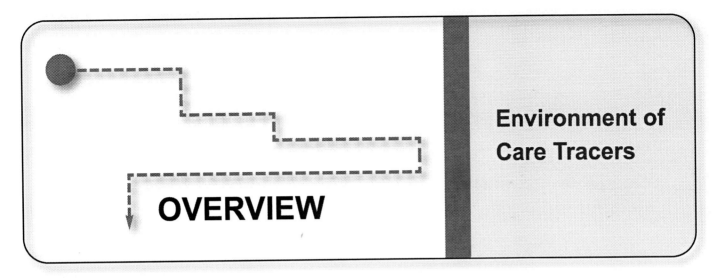

OVERVIEW

Environment of Care Tracers

As noted in the Introduction, tracers allow surveyors to assess organization systems and processes that drive care in the organization and affect the actual experiences of the individuals observed during the on-site evaluation.

Surveyors use the majority of their time on site performing tracers. During the tracers, surveyors assess how staff members from various disciplines work together to provide safe, high-quality care. Surveyors also talk with care recipients, when possible, to gain additional insight into their care experiences. These discussions with staff and individuals, combined with surveyors' review of documents and observations, make for a dynamic, interactive survey process.

Surveyors currently conduct individual tracers, system tracers, program-specific tracers, and environment of care (EC) tracers (which also include emergency management and life safety topics). EC tracers are similar to system tracers.

Tracers are not mutually exclusive. Information gathered during one type of tracer could play a part in issues explored during subsequent tracers. For example, surveyors could choose a system tracer or initiate an EC tracer based on observations or information gleaned during an individual tracer.

System Tracers

As noted previously, EC tracers are similar to system tracers. System tracer activity focuses on high-risk processes across organizations. The concept behind the system tracer methodology is to review processes at the organization. By examining a set of com-

ponents that work together toward a common goal, the surveyor can evaluate how and how well the organization's systems function.

System tracers provide a forum for discussing important topics related to the safety and quality of care, treatment, or services *at the organization level.* Surveyors use system tracers to examine organization findings and structure and to facilitate the exchange of educational information. Although some system tracer activities might consist of a more structured discussion between staff and surveyors, the processes depend on the size of the organization and the type of system tracer.

System Tracer Topics

A system tracer generally includes an interactive discussion between a surveyor and relevant staff members. Points of discussion can include the following:

- *Process flow:* The flow of the process through the organization, including identification and management of risk points, integration of key activities, and communication among staff and units involved in the process

- *Strengths and weaknesses:* Strengths in the process and possible actions to be taken in areas that need improvement

- *Issues to explore:* Issues requiring further exploration in other survey activities

- *Compliance:* A baseline assessment of standards compliance

- *Professional development:* Education by the surveyor, as appropriate

EC Tracers Plus EM and LS

As they do with all other standards, surveyors use tracer methodology to evaluate compliance with "Management of the Environment of Care" (EC) standards as well as with the "Emergency Management" (EM) and "Life Safety" (LS) standards. During the on-site survey of hospitals and critical access hospitals, a separate session is devoted to each of these areas: EC—the EC session; EM—the EM session; and LS—the *Life Safety Code®** building tour. (The other settings that receive a *Life Safety Code* building tour are ambulatory, behavioral health care, long term care, office based surgery, and facility-based home care settings.)

In addition, EC issues might come up during individual tracers as surveyors follow that care experience. (*See* the sidebar "Tracers at a Glance" in "How to Conduct a Mock Tracer" on page 6.)

The EC Session

In preparation for the EC session of an on-site survey, surveyors review the organization's annual evaluation of its EC management plans to become better oriented to the organization's environment. The EC session is divided between group discussion on managing risk in the organization's environment and performance of an EC tracer, during which the surveyor can observe and evaluate the organization's performance in managing EC risk.

During the discussion, the surveyor may explore the organization's risk assessment process and ask how the organization identifies potential risks. For example, the organization might use internal sources such as ongoing monitoring (EC.04.01.01), root cause analysis, or risk assessment of high-risk processes. The organization might also use credible external sources such as *Sentinel Event Alerts* (EC.02.01.01, EP 1, Note). The surveyor may request an example of a potential risk, the assessment process, and, if needed, the mitigation (*see* EC.02.01.01).

To close the EC session, surveyors and staff identify strengths and vulnerabilities in the environment and the actions necessary to address any vulnerabilities and assess the organization's compliance with relevant standards.

EC Risk Categories

Organizations can expect surveyors to trace a particular risk in one or more of the EC risk categories that the organization manages. The six EC risk categories are as follows:

- General safety
- Security
- Hazardous materials and waste
- Fire safety
- Medical/laboratory equipment (not applicable for behavioral health care)
- Utilities

In addition, of course, surveyors will be tracing EM and LS issues during the applicable survey sessions in the applicable health care settings. (See below for more information.)

Using the EC risk categories, the surveyor might begin where the potential risk is encountered or first occurs. It might be, for example, where a particular safety or security incident occurs, where a particular piece of medical equipment is used, or where a particular hazardous material enters the organization. The surveyor then talks with staff, asking them to describe or demonstrate their roles and responsibilities for minimizing the risk. In addition, the surveyor discusses with staff what they would do if a problem or an incident occurred and how they would report that problem or incident.

EM Session in Hospitals and Critical Access Hospitals

As of 2010, a separate EM session was added for hospitals and critical access hospitals. In preparation for this session, the surveyor reviews the Emergency Operations Plan (EOP), the hazard vulnerability analysis (HVA), and other EM–related documentation. This session is devoted to a discussion of the organization's EM activities. The surveyor concludes the session by summarizing the EM strengths and risks identified and how these might be explored in further individual tracers.

LS Tracers: The *Life Safety Code* Building Tour

In the case of settings such as ambulatory, behavioral health care, critical access hospitals, long term care, hospital, office-based surgery, and home care, a *Life Safety Code* building tour may be conducted by a *Life Safety Code* Specialist to assess the organization's compliance with key safety-issues. The *Life Safety Code* Specialist in effect "traces" the organization's compliance with the *Life Safety Code*, based on occupancy requirements.

---

*Life Safety Code is a registered trademark of the National Fire Protection Association, Quincy, MA.

Tracer Scenarios for
SAFETY

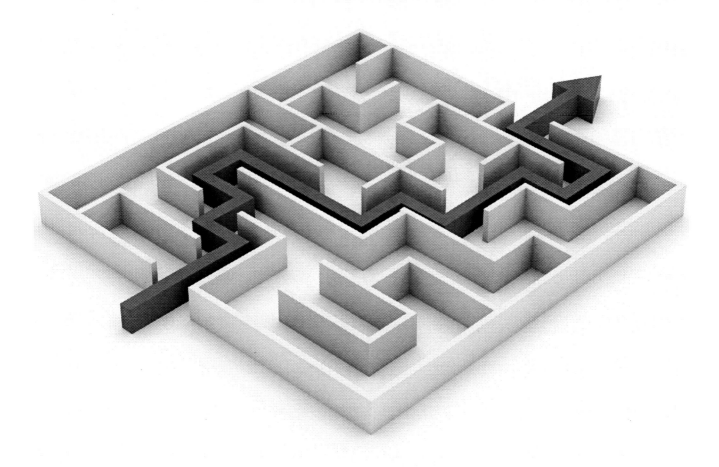

NOTE: No Two Tracers Are the Same

Please keep in mind that each tracer is unique. There is no way to know all of the questions that might be asked or documents that might be reviewed during a tracer—nor what all the responses to the questions and documents might be. The possibilities are limitless, depending on the tracer topic and the organization's circumstances. These tracer scenarios and sample questions are provided as an educational or training tool for organization staff; they are not scripts for real or mock tracers.

Section Elements

This section includes sample tracers—called scenarios—relevant to environmental safety. The section is organized as follows:

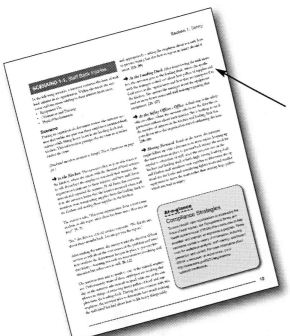

Scenarios: Each scenario presents what might happen when a surveyor conducts a specific type of tracer. The scenarios are presented in an engaging narrative format in which the reader "follows" the surveyor through the tracer scenario. Within the narrative are bracketed numbers that correspond to numbered sample tracer questions following the tracer.

Sample Tracer Questions: After each scenario narrative is a list of sample questions a surveyor might ask during that scenario. These questions can be used to develop and conduct mock tracers in your organization on topics similar to those covered in the scenario.

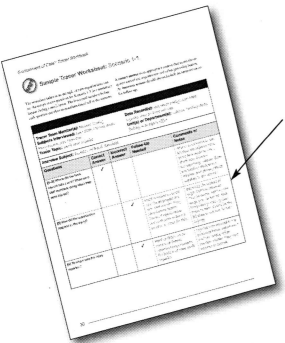

Sample Tracer Worksheet: At the end of the section is a sample worksheet that shows how the sample tracer questions for one select scenario in the section might be used in a worksheet format. The example shows how the worksheet might be completed as part of a tracer for that scenario. A blank form of the worksheet is available in Appendix B.

SCENARIO 1-1. Staff Back Injuries

In the following scenario, a surveyor examines the issue of staff back injuries in an organization. Within the tracer, the surveyor explores issues relating to these priority focus areas:

- Equipment Use
- Orientation and Training
- Physical Environment

Scenario

During an organization's document review, the surveyor notices that within the past year three employees sustained back injuries while lifting heavy items in the loading dock and kitchen. This information prompts the surveyor to examine further the issue.

(Bracketed numbers correlate to Sample Tracer Questions on page 20.)

➡ *In the Kitchen.* The surveyor's first stop on this tracer is the kitchen, where she meets with the director of food services to talk about how the employees sustained their injuries, the organization's response to those injuries, and how staff documented and reported the injuries. **[1–4]** From this conversation, the surveyor learns that the injuries occurred when staff members were transporting supplies from the loading dock to the kitchen and storing those supplies in the kitchen.

The surveyor asks, "Has your organization done a root cause analysis on this topic, since there has been more than one injury?" **[5–7]**

"Yes," the director of food services responds. "We did do one about three months back. Let me get you the report."

After reading the report, the surveyor asks the director of food services to talk about the root causes of the problem and what interventions the department has put in place to prevent further injury—focusing not only on interventions involving staff education but other ones as well. **[8–12]**

The surveyor then asks to speak to one of the injured employees. Unfortunately, none of these employees are working that day, so the surveyor asks instead to speak with one of the employees in charge of retrieving heavy pallets of food and supplies from the loading dock. During the conversation with this employee, the surveyor tries to determine how much training the individual has had about how to lift heavy things safely

and appropriately—asking the employee about not only how to prevent injury, but also how to report an injury should it occur. **[13–20]**

➡ *At the Loading Dock.* After interviewing the staff member, the surveyor goes to the loading dock, where she speaks with the manager to find out about how pallets of supplies and food arrive at the organization and how they are transported to the kitchen. She queries the manager about the equipment used to move heavy items and staff training regarding that equipment. **[21–27]**

➡ *At the Safety Officer's Office.* A final stop is the safety officer's office, where the surveyor asks to see the data the organization collects about back injuries. She is looking to see if the number of injuries in the kitchen and loading dock has gone down since the organization started addressing the issue. **[28–30]**

➡ *Moving Forward.* Based on the tracer, the surveyor might follow up with a discussion on these topics: keeping up the interventions in place to prevent back injury; the need for regular re-education of staff, since the turnover rate in the kitchen and loading dock is fairly high; having loading dock and kitchen staff members work together to determine the optimal size for loads; and considering lighter loads and smaller equipment to move the loads rather than moving large pallets, which can lead to injury.

At-a-glance
Compliance Strategies

To assist health care organizations in addressing the issue of back injuries, the Occupational Safety and Health Administration (OSHA) offers resources to help establish and maintain an ergonomics program. These resources contain a variety of information, including tools for workplace analysis, staff training, and hazard prevention and control. For more information about OSHA's resources on ergonomics, go to http://www.osha.gov/SLTC/ergonomics/outreach.html#etools.

MOCK TRACER TIP

An organization may be experiencing employee injuries in other areas besides the kitchen and loading dock, such as within patient care units, areas housing heavy equipment, and housekeeping locations. When considering where to perform a mock tracer related to employee injury, an organization should review its data and think about performing the mock tracer in the area that has the highest injury rate.

Scenario 1-1.
Sample Tracer Questions

The bracketed numbers before each question correlate to questions, observations, and data review described in the sample tracer for Scenario 1-1. You can use the tracer worksheet form in Appendix B to develop a mock tracer (*see* an example of a completed tracer worksheet at the end of this section). The information gained by conducting a mock tracer can help to highlight a good practice and/or determine issues that may require further follow-up.

Director of Food Services

[1]   Where did the back injuries take place?

[2]   What were staff members doing when they were injured?

[3]   How did the organization respond to the injury?

[4]   To whom was the injury reported?

[5]   Did the organization conduct a root cause analysis?

[6]   Who was involved in the root cause analysis?

[7]   What did the organization determine to be the root causes of the problem?

[8]   What solutions did the organization put in place to prevent this type of injury in the future?

[9]   What has the organization done, besides re-educate staff, to make things safer?

[10]   Has the organization seen improvement as a result of its efforts?

[11]   How did the organization educate staff on preventing back injuries?

[12]   How often does the organization re-educate staff on this topic?

Kitchen Employee

[13]   What do you do when lifting pallets of supplies to prevent injury?

[14]   Show me how you would lift something heavy.

[15]   What are the risks of lifting something in an inappropriate way?

[16]   If you sustain an injury lifting something, what do you do?

[17]   Who do you notify?

[18]   Do you feel the organization creates a safe environment in which you can work?

[19]   What education have you received on how to prevent back injuries?

[20]   Do you think you need more education on this topic?

Loading Dock Manager

[21]   How are pallets removed from the loading dock?

[22]   What equipment is used?

[23]   Are staff members trained to use the equipment?

[24]   Do staff members have to do heavy lifting to remove the pallet?

[25]   Are staff members trained on how to lift properly?

[26]   How does the organization determine how much a staff member can lift?

[27]   Is there a limit to the amount of weight a staff member is permitted to lift?

Safety Officer

[28]   How often does the organization review employee injury data?

[29]   Who is in charge of reviewing those data?

[30]   Has the number of employee back injuries gone down since the organization performed the root cause analysis and implemented interventions?

SCENARIO 1-2. Patient Falls

Summary

In the following scenario, a surveyor examines the topic of patient falls. Within the tracer, the surveyor explores issues relating to these priority focus areas:

- Assessment and Care Services
- Communication
- Equipment Use
- Orientation and Training
- Patient Safety
- Physical Environment

Scenario

A surveyor is up on patient care unit 5E, tracing the care of an elderly patient who is at risk for falling. During the course of the tracer, the surveyor asks to see the unit's data on patient falls. Upon reviewing the data, he notices that the unit has a higher-than-expected fall rate. This prompts the surveyor to examine further the issue.

(Bracketed numbers correlate to Sample Tracer Questions on pages 22–23.)

➡ ***At the Patient Care Unit.*** The surveyor begins his exploration by speaking with the nurse who is working with the elderly patient. The surveyor asks the nurse about the processes for assessing fall risk, the procedures to respond to a patient who has been determined to be at risk for falls, and the interventions used to prevent falls. **[1–2]**

"What environmental controls does this unit have to prevent falls?" the surveyor asks. "Well, the floors have a nonskid surface on them, and we have handrails positioned throughout the unit," the nurse responds. "In addition, we are pretty scrupulous about lighting. It's important that the hallways, bathrooms, patient rooms, and so on are well lit, so patients can see where they're going. Our maintenance department is really good about keeping all the lightbulbs fresh." **[3]**

The surveyor chats with the nurse about how she uses technology—such as assistive devices and wheelchair alarms—to prevent falls. **[4–5]**

After talking with the nurse, the surveyor stands aside and watches her work with the elderly patient. He notes how the nurse uses preventive and assistive technology, communicates with other providers about the patient's fall risk, and responds to a spill on the floor that could present a slipping hazard.

The surveyor then takes a closer look at the unit itself. He notices some loose floor tiles that could present a tripping hazard. He also observes that part of the floor surface is somewhat slick and that the shoes that staff members are wearing may put *them* at risk for falls.

After observing the staff member and the unit, the surveyor approaches another nurse and asks him what he would do if a patient fell, including how he would respond to the patient, how he would report the issue, and what the next steps would be to prevent this type of incident from happening again. **[6–8]** The surveyor also speaks with the nurse about any training and education he has received regarding fall prevention, including how to assess for falls, use interventions to prevent falls, and respond to falls. **[9]**

"How much training have you had about fall prevention?" asks the surveyor. The nurse responds, "We just did an in-service a couple months ago, and the supervisor is always posting information sheets around the unit about being aware of patient fall risk. We are supposed to get some new equipment in the next few months. I am sure we'll get some training when that arrives."

Finally, the surveyor asks the nurse if he is aware of his own risk for falling and whether he knows how to prevent falls for himself. **[10–11]**

The surveyor then spends some time talking with the manager of the unit. He asks about the training offered for staff, how often that training is provided, and what processes are in place for fall prevention and response. **[12–14]** The surveyor's goal here is to make sure that the staff members' responses mirror the manager's responses.

> ### MOCK TRACER TIP
>
> Although this tracer stemmed from reviewing data about a particular unit's fall rate, organizations can also identify areas at risk for employee and visitor falls by looking at employee health records, minutes of the environment of care (EC) safety committee, and OSHA reporting documentation. Once an area of risk is identified, an organization can use a tracer to help explore compliance issues in that area.

➡ *Talking with Transport Staff.* After speaking with the manager, the surveyor asks to talk with a transport staff member. He is introduced to a young man who has been transporting patients in the organization for six months. The surveyor asks how the staff member prevents falls during patient transport. Just as with direct care staff, the surveyor asks about responding to a patient fall, documenting a patient fall, and training and education. **[15–18]** During this conversation, the transport staff member mentions that he saw a patient fall recently in the diagnostic testing area. The surveyor asks him to describe the incident and then asks the staff member to take him to the area where the fall occurred.

➡ *At the Diagnostic Testing Area.* In the diagnostic testing area, the surveyor observes the area for a few minutes, watching to see how transport staff communicate with diagnostic testing area personnel about patients identified as being at risk of falling, the use of environmental controls for fall risk, and the use of assistive devices. The surveyor then speaks with diagnostic testing personnel about how they are informed of a patient's risk for falling and what they do with that information. He probes for information about the processes in place in the area for preventing and responding to patient falls during testing. He also talks with staff members about orientation and training. **[15–18]** Finally, he observes the unit for any environmental contributors to fall risk.

➡ *Consulting with the Safety Officer.* Before concluding the tracer, the surveyor makes a brief stop at the office of the safety officer. He asks to see the notes from the most recent environmental tours and checks to see if the organization is looking for potential fall risks during these tours. He queries the safety officer about how the organization responds to any identified fall risks—specifically focusing on the fall risks on 5E. **[19–21]**

➡ *Moving Forward.* Based on the tracer, the surveyor might follow up with a discussion on these topics: performing a root cause analysis for falls on 5E and within the diagnostic testing area, since although the organization has some good processes in place, its fall rate indicates that it could be doing more to prevent patient falls, and incorporating more environmental controls to help ensure that the environment does not exacerbate fall risks for patients.

At-a-glance
Compliance Strategies

The best way to identify environmental fall risk factors in an organization is to conduct an environmental assessment. Some areas to examine within this assessment include the following:

- Lighting in patient areas and hallways
- Degree of clutter and obstructions in patient walkways
- Stability of handrails
- Sturdiness of furniture
- Security of locks and window openings
- Safety of equipment such as assistive devices, alarms, call bells, beds, and so forth
- Hazards in the outside terrain

Scenario 1-2.
Sample Tracer Questions

The bracketed numbers before each question correlate to questions, observations, and data review described in the sample tracer for Scenario 1-2. You can use the tracer worksheet form in Appendix B to develop a mock tracer (*see* an example of a completed tracer worksheet at the end of this section). The information gained by conducting a mock tracer can help to highlight a good practice and/or determine issues that may require further follow-up.

Direct Care Staff

[1] What is the process for assessing a patient for fall risk?

[2] What do you do when the process shows that a patient is at risk for falling?

[3] What environmental controls does the organization have in place to prevent falls?

[4] What technology (such as assistive devices) does the organization use to prevent falls?

[5] What do you do if that technology fails?

[6] How do you respond if a patient falls?

[7] How is the fall reported?

[8] What do you do to prevent falls in the future?

[9] What orientation and training have you received regarding fall prevention?

[10] Are you aware of how to prevent yourself from falling?

[11] What do you do when you see an environmental risk for falls, such as a spill?

Unit Manager

[12] What is the department's orientation and training for falls?

[13] How often is that training provided?

[14] What do you as a manager do to prevent patient and employee falls?

Transport and Diagnostic Testing Staff

[15] How are you informed that a patient is at risk for falls?

[16] What is the process for preventing a fall during transport?

[17] How do you respond when a patient falls?

[18] What orientation and training do you receive regarding fall prevention?

Safety Officer

[19] Does the organization examine environmental risks regarding falls during environmental tours?

[20] What do you do when you discover an environmental risk?

[21] Has the organization done a root cause analysis on environmental risks for falls?

SCENARIO 1-3. Snow Removal

Summary

In the following scenario, a surveyor at a Midwestern organization conducts a tracer about snow removal. Within the tracer, the surveyor explores issues relating to these priority focus areas:

- Communication
- Patient Safety
- Physical Environment
- Staffing

Scenario

Light snow is falling as a surveyor enters a Midwestern organization on the first day of its triennial survey. But by noon that day, the snow showers of the morning have turned into a more serious snowfall, with accumulation up to 3 inches. The weather forecast predicts another 6 inches of snow by midnight.

As part of the organization's EC session, the surveyor decides to examine the organization's processes for snow removal, focusing specifically on how the organization ensures that its outside pathways—sidewalks, parking lots, and other walkways—are kept safe.

(Bracketed numbers correlate to Sample Tracer Questions on pages 24–25.)

➡ *A Tour of Walkways.* The surveyor begins the tracer by asking the director of facilities and the safety officer to join him on a tour of the external walkways and parking lot. As they tour the area, the surveyor takes note of how clean the sidewalks are, whether there are any tripping hazards, and whether slippery areas are clearly indicated with signage.

➡ *At the Main Entrance.* At the main entrance to the facility, the surveyor stops and observes patients, visitors, and staff entering and exiting the building to see if anyone has any problems traversing the sidewalks outside the building and the walkways into the building.

While the surveyor observes the pedestrians, he chats with the director of facilities and the safety officer, asking them about the organization's processes for managing snow removal, using salt, and maintaining slip-free surfaces. **[1–8]** He is attempting to determine whether the organization has a specific approach to snow removal or whether it is haphazard.

➡ *A Conversation with a Maintenance Worker.* After observing patients, visitors, and staff enter and exit the building, the surveyor approaches a maintenance worker who is removing snow from one of the sidewalks and asks if he may talk with her about snow removal. **[10–14]** The surveyor wants to see if the maintenance worker's perspective on the importance

MOCK TRACER TIP

With a topic like snow removal, it is critical not to just talk about the safety issues but to observe how the organization ensures safety during inclement weather. The key element in this tracer is actually watching people enter and exit the building. Talking to an individual who is working on removing the snow is also important because the person doing the tracer is interacting with the maintenance individual as he or she is doing the work.

of removing snow mirrors that of the organization. In addition, the surveyor wants to learn whether the maintenance worker understands her responsibilities and the responsibilities of her coworkers in ensuring the safety of patients, staff, and visitors who enter and exit the facility.

During the conversation, the surveyor notices that there is no signage present in the area. "Tell me, do you have signs that warn patients and visitors that an area is potentially slippery?" asks the surveyor. **[15–17]** "Yes, we have those, but we usually use them inside and not outside," responds the maintenance employee. "In fact, we are pretty short on signs today because the snow has created many slippery areas. We don't have

At-a-glance
Compliance Strategies

Conducting environmental tours is an excellent way for an organization to identify safety risks—including those related to inclement weather. These tours can help reveal environmental deficiencies, hazardous conditions, and unsafe practices. Environmental tours involve more than someone walking around, pointing out things that are potentially unsafe. Rather, the tours are multidisciplinary exercises through which an organization can observe safety practices and behaviors, eliminate potential hazards, and monitor staff knowledge in an effort to maintain a safe environment for patients, visitors, and staff. During tours, an organization can also determine whether it is practicing and enforcing its safety policies and procedures and effectively managing its safety risks.

To streamline the process of environmental tours, an organization may want to create a checklist. This helps avoid overlooking or forgetting particular areas. Each member of the team participating in the tour should have a copy of the checklist to fill out during the tour. Different team members can be in charge of filling out different sections of the checklist, as appropriate. The individual in charge of the tour process should review all checklist forms and might want to merge all identified issues onto one form. This will prevent duplication of information and also ensure that every issue is documented.

enough signs to go around. So, we put signs where we think there is the biggest chance someone might slip."

➡️ *A Data Review.* After the surveyor speaks to the maintenance worker, he asks the director of facilities and the safety officer, "By the way, do you have any data on visitor falls—specifically those falls related to the weather?" **[9]** "Yes, we have those data," says the director of facilities. "We keep the data in my office and review them every six months."

After returning to the office of the director of facilities, the surveyor reviews the data and notes that there is a higher percentage of falls at the north entrance than in other locations. After a brief discussion, the surveyor and the director of facilities determine that because the north entrance does not receive any direct sunlight, it takes longer for ice and snow to melt from the area. The surveyor recommends that the organization consider increasing its attention to that area as well as ensuring proper signage.

➡️ *Moving Forward.* Based on the tracer, the surveyor might follow up with a discussion on these topics: reviewing procedures regarding snow removal to develop a more responsive approach; using security cameras to help monitor exits and sidewalks—particularly problem areas—during inclement weather to see clearly whether people are having difficulty traversing particular areas; and purchasing more signs and developing a process to ensure that appropriate signage is posted during slippery conditions.

Scenario 1-3.
Sample Tracer Questions

The bracketed numbers before each question correlate to questions, observations, and data review described in the sample tracer for Scenario 1-3. You can use the tracer worksheet form in Appendix B to develop a mock tracer (*see* an example of a completed tracer worksheet at the end of this section). The information gained by conducting a mock tracer can help to highlight a good practice and/or determine issues that may require further follow-up.

Director of Facilities/Safety Officer

[1] What are the organization's processes for managing snow removal?

[2] Does the organization use salt? If so, how does the organization determine how much salt to use?

[3] Are staff members given protective gear to prevent salt from causing skin-related issues?

[4] How does the organization keep up with snow removal during a snowstorm?

[5] How many staff members are dedicated to snow removal? Does this change depending on the weather conditions?

[6] How do staff members know when they are needed for snow removal?

[7] Do staff members receive training regarding snow removal?

[8] What does the organization do when inclement weather is predicted? Does it call in reserve staff? Is there a system for this? If so, describe it.

[9] Does the organization monitor data regarding falls related to inclement weather? If so, what has the organization discovered?

Maintenance Worker

[10] What do you do when snow is predicted?

[11] What do you do when snow begins to fall?

[12] Does the organization have adequate equipment for snow removal?

[13] Where is that equipment stored? Is it easy to access?

[14] Do you know how to use that equipment? If so, did you learn this through training or by some other means?

[15] Does the organization have signs that point out potentially slippery areas?

[16] Do you think there are enough signs? Why or why not?

[17] What is the process for distributing these signs?

SCENARIO 1-4. Eyewash Stations

Summary

In the following scenario, a surveyor traces the safety and maintenance of an organization's eyewash stations. Within the tracer, the surveyor explores issues relating to these priority focus areas:

- Equipment Use
- Orientation and Training
- Physical Environment

Scenario

When reviewing the minutes of an organization's EC commit-tee meetings, a surveyor notes that the organization recently installed some new eyewash stations in and around its pharmacy and laboratory. The surveyor decides to trace the placement, use, and maintenance of these eyewash stations.

(Bracketed numbers correlate to Sample Tracer Questions on pages 26–27.)

→ *At the Pharmacy.* The surveyor's first stop is the pharmacy, where she observes the location of the new eyewash stations. She looks to see if the stations are located appropriately, with clear and unobstructed access. She then introduces herself to the pharmacy manager and asks how the new eyewash stations are working out. She explores whether they have been used, and if they have been, how that went. **[1–2]**

"Has there been any training and education on these eyewash stations?" asks the surveyor. "Yes," responds the manager. "The manufacturer provided some written material on the stations, and we developed that into a PowerPoint presentation that I gave at the most recent staff meeting. We also keep an at-a-glance fact sheet posted by each station." **[3]**

The surveyor and manager then discuss training and education about responding to chemical splashes involving the eye and how to report any incidents involving the eyewash stations. **[4]**

Following this conversation, the surveyor requests the testing records for the eyewash stations, and, after reviewing the records, asks to speak with the individual in charge of testing the stations. **[5–6]**

"How do you test these eyewash stations?" the surveyor asks. "I run each one for about 12 minutes every Friday during the lunch hour, because most of the pharmacy staff are out of the pharmacy at that time," says the employee. "Once I run the test, I document it on a maintenance log next to the station." **[7–11]**

MOCK TRACER TIP

For some organizations, the maintenance department will be charged with testing eyewash stations. To verify that testing activities in these cases are occurring appropriately and on schedule, an organization should visit the maintenance department and trace how it tests eyewash stations and how it documents that testing.

"How hot is the water in the stations?" asks the surveyor. **[12]** "The stations use tepid water, because hot water can exacerbate an injury," says the employee. "We know the water is tepid because of the mixing valve on the station that helps ensure the proper water temperature."

Next, the surveyor approaches a pharmacist and asks if she can speak with her about the eyewash stations. During this conversation, the surveyor gathers information about the pharmacist's familiarity with the location of the stations, when to use the stations, and how to use them. She also asks the pharmacist what training she has received on the eyewash stations specifically, as well as on how to respond to a chemical splash in general. **[13–20]**

➡ **At the Laboratory.** After visiting the pharmacy, the surveyor goes to the laboratory, where she talks about the eyewash stations with the laboratory manager. [1–4] After this conversation, she passes a laboratory staff member who is working with a hazardous liquid. She stops and asks the employee what he would do if that liquid splashed in his eyes. This discussion focuses on not only how he would use the eyewash station but where he would go after using the eyewash station. "I would go to the emergency department (ED) for further treatment," responds the employee. **[13–20]**

➡ **At the ED.** The next stop is the ED, where the surveyor asks a nurse how she would respond if an employee arrived in the ED after being splashed in the eye with a hazardous chemical. This conversation focuses on not only the steps involved in treating the employee but how long the employee could expect to wait before receiving treatment. **[21–23]**

At-a-glance
Compliance Strategies

Although having readily accessible eyewash stations is key to employee safety, using personal protective equipment (PPE) for the face—including eye masks, goggles, and face shields—is the number-one defense against chemical splashes. Such equipment should be worn when splashing is reasonably anticipated, and staff should be familiar with how to use such equipment and why it is important.

➡ *Moving Forward.* Based on the tracer, the surveyor might follow up with a discussion on developing a continuing emphasis on staff training, not only regarding the eyewash stations but also concerning how to respond to and get treatment for a chemical splash that affects the eyes.

Scenario 1-4.
Sample Tracer Questions

The bracketed numbers before each question correlate to questions, observations, and data review described in the sample tracer for Scenario 1-4. You can use the tracer worksheet form in Appendix B to develop a mock tracer (*see* an example of a completed tracer worksheet at the end of this section). The information gained by conducting a mock tracer can help to highlight a good practice and/or determine issues that may require further follow-up.

Pharmacy/Laboratory Manager

[1] How long has the organization had the new eyewash stations?

[2] Has there been an incident in which the eyewash stations were used? Describe that incident.

[3] What training does the department provide on the eyewash stations? What training does the department provide on responding to a chemical splash?

[4] How do you report an incident involving the eyewash stations?

[5] Where do you keep testing records for the eyewash stations?

[6] Who is responsible for testing the eyewash stations?

Pharmacy Technician

[7] How do you test the eyewash stations?

[8] How often do you test them?

[9] How do you document this testing?

[10] What do you do when the testing shows that an eyewash station is not functioning properly?

[11] Who do you contact to fix the eyewash station?

[12] How hot is the water in the stations?

Pharmacist/Laboratory Employee

[13] What PPE equipment do you wear to protect your eyes from chemical splashes?

[14] Why is it important to wear this equipment?

[15] What would you do if you splashed a hazardous chemical in your eye?

[16] Describe where the eyewash stations are located.

[17] What training have you had on the new eyewash stations?

[18] What training have you had on the proper response to a chemical splash?

[19] What are the risks involved in splashing chemicals?

[20] If a chemical splashes in your eye, where would you go after using the eyewash station?

ED Nurse

[21] How would you treat an employee who came to the ED after splashing a chemical in his or her eyes?

[22] How quickly would that employee receive treatment?

[23] Would treating that employee be a priority?

SCENARIO 1-5. Elevator Safety

Summary

In the following scenario, a surveyor traces the safety and maintenance of an organization's elevators. Within the tracer, the surveyor explores issues relating to these priority focus areas:

- Equipment Use
- Physical Environment

Scenario

As a surveyor enters a long term care organization to conduct its triennial survey, he spots a repair person working on one of the elevators. He stops to chat with the contractor, asking him about his work at the organization and why he was called to fix the elevator. The repair person indicates that there was an elevator stoppage last week, and a patient and nurse were stuck in the elevator for about an hour. He is on site to do some troubleshooting to figure out what happened. Curious about the incident, the surveyor decides to trace the safety of the organization's elevators.

(Bracketed numbers correlate to Sample Tracer Questions on pages 28–29.)

➡ *At the Facility Manager's Office.* During this tracer, the surveyor first stops in at the facility manager's office, asking about the elevators and their history. He requests the maintenance logs and spends some time reviewing them. He notes that an outside company tests and services the elevators regularly. All appears to be in order. However, it comes up in conversation with the facility manager that this is the fourth time this particular elevator—called E1—has malfunctioned in the past year. **[1–4]**

➡ *At the Elevator.* After their initial conversation, the facility manager walks the surveyor to the bank of elevators, where the surveyor observes their condition. The surveyor takes a ride on an elevator, stopping at every floor to make sure the doors open properly and the ride is smooth. He checks the flooring to make sure it doesn't present a tripping hazard and also looks at the lighting to make sure it is adequate for the space.

During this time, the surveyor chats further with the facility manager about the incidents in which E1 stopped. The surveyor probes for information about what happened, why it happened, and whether the facility manager feels is was a pattern. **[5–7]**

"How did you know the elevator was stuck?" asks the surveyor. **[8–10]** "When the elevator stopped, I could hear the alarm, and then the nurse in the elevator picked up the emergency phone, which is directly connected to my office phone. I was able to reassure the nurse that everything would be okay, and we were working on the problem. She and I remained on the line until the elevator resumed service."

The surveyor then probes about the duration of the elevator outage and how the elevator was fixed. **[11–12]**

➡ *At the Nurses' Station.* After speaking with the facility manager, the surveyor asks to chat with the patient and nurse who were stuck in the elevator. He first visits the nurse. During this conversation, the surveyor tries to determine what the nurse did when the elevator stopped working. He wants to find out who she contacted, how she contacted that person, and how she kept the patient calm. In this conversation, he is looking to see that the nurse's responses mirror those of the facility manager. **[16–21]**

"Do you think this elevator outage represents a pattern of which the organization should be aware?" asks the surveyor. **[22–23]** "Well, it certainly doesn't happen all the time, but I will admit I am a bit concerned when I get into that elevator now, because it is known to malfunction," says the nurse.

"Mine was not the only incident. With that said, I know the facilities manager is working on the issue and is taking my concerns as well as other people's seriously."

➡ ***In the Patient's Room.*** The surveyor spends some time with the patient who was stuck in E1, asking her about her experience. The patient indicates that the nurse was very good about remaining calm and that the facility manager was on the phone with the nurse the whole time the elevator was stuck. Although she was a little nervous and was happy when the elevator started working again, the patient thought the staff handled the incident very well. She also mentions that she's seen several people working on the elevator since the incident, so she knows the organization is taking what happened seriously. **[24–28]**

➡ ***At the Facility Manager's Office.*** The surveyor returns to the facility manager's office for one more conversation. He wants to determine what the organization is doing to prevent an occurrence like this from happening again. Although it has not been a weekly event, the elevator has stopped more than

once in the past year, and if it stops while it has a critical patient on board, the consequences could be serious. The surveyor asks whether the organization has done a root cause analysis and, if so, what the results of that analysis were. **[13–15]** The facility manager indicates that the organization has brought repair personnel from the elevator manufacturer to the organization to check the elevators, but a complete root cause analysis has not been done.

➡ ***Moving Forward.*** Based on the tracer, the surveyor might follow up with a discussion on engaging in a root cause analysis of the elevator problem—and ideally including the manufacturer in the exercise as well as getting organization leadership on board because any large-scale improvements to the elevator might involve a capital expenditure.

MOCK TRACER TIP

During tracers involving contracted services—such as the elevator repair person—it can be helpful to speak with the individual actually providing the contracted services, if possible. Although talking with a company representative—such as a sales person—can also provide insight, the most benefit comes from actually speaking to someone who is doing the work.

At-a-glance
Compliance Strategies

Safety issues may be present in elevators because of the mechanical operation of the elevators as well as their flooring, ceiling construction, and lighting. In addition, elevators present the possibility of comingling clean and soiled items, which should be avoided. Including the elevators on environmental tours can help ensure that an organization quickly discovers potential safety issues concerning the elevators.

Scenario 1-5.
Sample Tracer Questions

The bracketed numbers before each question correlate to questions, observations, and data review described in the sample tracer for Scenario 1-5. You can use the tracer worksheet form in Appendix B to develop a mock tracer (*see* an example of a completed tracer worksheet at the end of this section). The information gained by conducting a mock tracer can help to highlight a good practice and/or determine issues that may require further follow-up.

Facility Manager

[1]   How old are the elevators in this building?

[2]   How well do the elevators perform?

[3]   Does the organization do regular maintenance on them?

[4]   Can I see the maintenance records?

[5]   Describe the elevator failure incident.

[6]   Why do you think the elevator stopped?

[7]   Do you think this is a pattern?

[8]   How were you notified of the failure?

[9]   How did you communicate with the occupants of the elevator?

[10] How did you ensure that the occupants of the elevator remained calm?

[11] Who did you call to fix the elevator?

[12] How quickly were you able to get the elevator working?

[13] What is the organization doing to prevent this occurrence from happening again?

[14] Has the organization done a root cause analysis on this issue?

[15] What are the results of that analysis?

Nurse on the Unit

[16] What did you do when the elevator stopped?

[17] Who did you notify?

[18] Were the systems of notification working?

[19] Were you comfortable with how to use the systems of notification?

[20] How did you keep the patient calm?

[21] Were you ever concerned about your safety or the patient's safety?

[22] Do you think this elevator failure represents a pattern?

[23] Do you think the organization is addressing the issue?

Patient

[24] How did you feel when the elevator stopped?

[25] Did the nurse react in a professional manner?

[26] Did the nurse stay in contact with someone outside the elevator?

[27] Did you feel that you were safe?

[28] Do you think the organization is addressing the problem?

Sample Tracer Worksheet: Scenario 1-1.

The worksheet below is an example of how organizations can use the sample tracer questions for Scenario 1-1 in a worksheet format during a mock tracer. The bracketed numbers before each question correlate to questions described in the scenario.

A **correct answer** is an appropriate answer that meets the requirements of the organization and other governing bodies. An **incorrect answer** should always include recommendations for follow-up.

Tracer Team Member(s): Darlene Quealy
Subjects Interviewed: Jan Leitch, Marcus Jones, Tony Rivera, Jack Thornton
Tracer Topic: Staff back injuries

Data Record(s): OSHA 300 log; root cause analysis on back injuries
Unit(s) or Department(s): Kitchen, loading dock, facility manager's office

Interview Subject: Director of Food Services

Questions	Correct Answer	Incorrect Answer	Follow-Up Needed	Comments or Notes
[1–2] Where did the back injuries take place? What were staff members doing when they were injured?	✓			Able to show where in the kitchen the injuries took place and describe what staff were doing—transporting supplies from the loading dock to the kitchen and storing those supplies in the kitchen
[3] How did the organization respond to the injury?		✓	Need to follow up to see how the employees are now and whether they have further health issues. Organization does not seem to have a process in place for this.	Describes the process of organization response. This includes treating the employees in the ED and temporarily reassigning them to other duties in the kitchen to prevent further injury.
[4] To whom was the injury reported?		✓	Need to follow up on state and federal reporting requirements for back and other staff injuries.	Injuries were reported to the employee health department and the safety office. Unclear whether they were reported to OSHA.

Interview Subject: Director of Food Services (continued)				
Questions	**Correct Answer**	**Incorrect Answer**	**Follow-Up Needed**	**Comments or Notes**
[5] Did the organization conduct a root cause analysis?	✓			Root cause analysis (RCA) was timely and looked at the reasons behind the recurrent injuries. Examined the report generated by the RCA. It appears thorough and well considered.
[6] Who was involved in the root cause analysis?		✓	Suggest involving senior leadership in some fashion. While they don't have to fully participate in the RCA, they should be aware of the activity, so as to know that back injury is an issue for the organization.	Team members included: Director of food service, loading dock manager, safety officer, facilities manager, kitchen employee, loading dock employee.
[7] What did the organization determine to be the root causes of the problem?	✓			Able to describe root causes in some detail—inconsistent education, poor communication, need to get supplies in a hurry, so staff rush through transport.
[8–9] What solutions did the organization put in place to prevent this type of injury in the future? What has the organization done, besides re-educate staff, to make things safer?	✓		Loading dock and kitchen staff should work together to determine optimal loads.	Increased education to employees, tested new equipment for transporting pallets, provided staff with back belts, observed staff, and gave just-in-time training about proper lifting.
[10] Has the organization seen improvement as a result of its efforts?		✓	Organization needs to work on measuring improvements.	No definitive system in place for measuring success.

(continued)

Interview Subject: Director of Food Services (continued)

Questions	Correct Answer	Incorrect Answer	Follow-Up Needed	Comments or Notes
[11] How did the organization educate staff on preventing back injuries?		✓	Need to follow up on this training to see if it was effective. Perhaps by observing staff? Asking staff about appropriate lifting during environmental tours?	Provided in-services, just-in-time training, and access to online video. No way to know if these are successful.
[12] How often does the organization re-educate staff on this topic?		✓	May want to develop a more regular schedule of training or include this topic in currently scheduled training.	Part of new staff orientation. Also some training for staff throughout the year. Done on an ad hoc basis.

Interview Subject: Kitchen Employee

Questions	Correct Answer	Incorrect Answer	Follow-Up Needed	Comments or Notes
[13–14] What do you do when lifting pallets of supplies to prevent injury? Show me how you would lift something heavy.	✓			Able to describe the appropriate way to lift a heavy object, including a pallet.
[15] What are the risks of lifting something in an inappropriate way?		✓	Need to work with staff to understand the risks involved in heavy lifting and the consequences of lifting in an inappropriate way.	Does not seem clear on the degree of risk involved in lifting heavy objects. He knows he could hurt himself but doesn't realize that injury could result in chronic back problems and ultimately affect job performance.
[16–17] If you sustain an injury lifting something, what do you do? Who do you notify?	✓		Need to work with staff on how to follow up after an incident if an injury flares up.	Staff member is clear on where to report injury and to whom. Also knows to visit the ED. Seems a little unsure about how to follow up if the injury does not present itself until later.

Interview Subject: Kitchen Employee (continued)

Questions	Correct Answer	Incorrect Answer	Follow-Up Needed	Comments or Notes
[18] Do you feel the organization creates a safe environment in which you can work?	✓			Indicates he felt safe at work. Thinks the organization cares about his well-being.
[19–20] What education have you received on how to prevent back injuries? Do you think you need more education on this topic?		✓	As mentioned previously, should work on providing training within a more regular schedule.	Describes varied education opportunities. Definitely ad hoc in nature.

Interview Subject: Loading Dock Manager

Questions	Correct Answer	Incorrect Answer	Follow-Up Needed	Comments or Notes
[21–22] How are pallets removed from the loading dock? What equipment is used?		✓	May want to look at this process to see if it can be improved.	Manager able to describe specific process.
[23–25] Are staff members trained to use the equipment? to lift properly? Do they have to do heavy lifting?		✓	See above.	Describes several good training opportunities. Again, ad hoc.
[26–27] How does the organization determine how much a staff member can lift? Is there a limit to the amount of weight is permitted to lift?		✓	Should spend time determining a way to figure out how much a staff member is allowed to lift.	No processes for determining appropriate weight for lifting.

Interview Subject: Director of Facilities

Questions	Correct Answer	Incorrect Answer	Follow-Up Needed	Comments or Notes
[28–30] How often does the organization review employee injury data? Who is in charge of this review? Has the number of employee back injuries gone down since the organization performed the root cause analysis and implemented interventions?		✓	Should define a time frame for injury review and stick with it.	Cannot articulate a specific time frame in which he reviews injury data. Seems haphazard.

Tracer Scenarios for
SECURITY

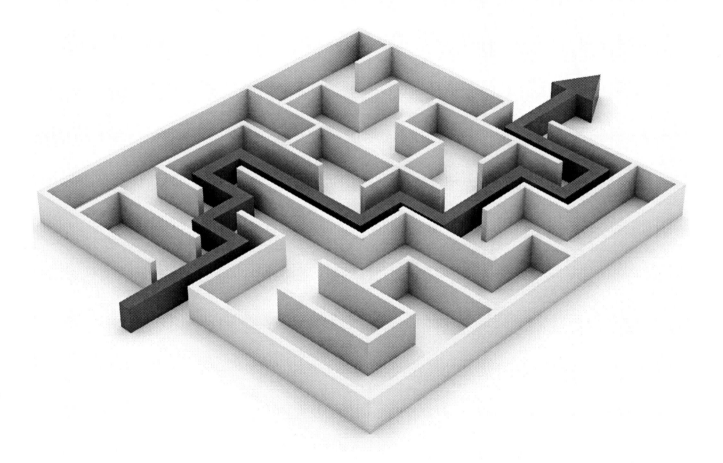

NOTE: No Two Tracers Are the Same

Please keep in mind that each tracer is unique. There is no way to know all of the questions that might be asked or documents that might be reviewed during a tracer—or what all the responses to the questions and documents might be. The possibilities are limitless, depending on the tracer topic and the organization's circumstances. These tracer scenarios and sample questions are provided as educational or training tools for organization staff; they are not scripts for real or mock tracers.

Section Elements

This section includes sample tracers—called scenarios—relevant to organization security. The section is organized as follows:

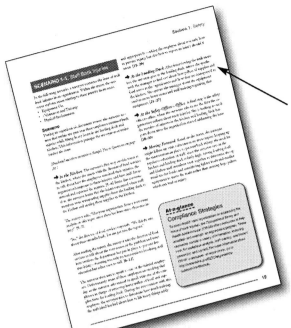

Scenarios: Each scenario presents what might happen when a surveyor conducts a specific type of tracer. The scenarios are presented in an engaging narrative format in which the reader "follows" the surveyor through the tracer scenario. Within the narrative are bracketed numbers that correspond to numbered sample tracer questions following the tracer.

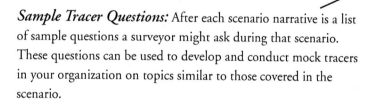

Sample Tracer Questions: After each scenario narrative is a list of sample questions a surveyor might ask during that scenario. These questions can be used to develop and conduct mock tracers in your organization on topics similar to those covered in the scenario.

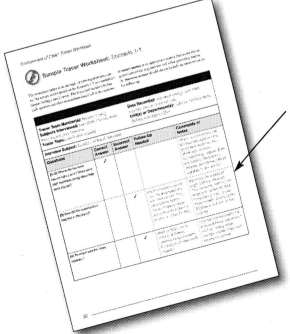

Sample Tracer Worksheet: At the end of the section is a sample worksheet that shows how the sample tracer questions for one select scenario in the section might be used in a worksheet format. The example shows how the worksheet might be completed as part of a tracer for that scenario. A blank form of the worksheet is available in Appendix B.

SCENARIO 2-1. Infant and Pediatric Security

Summary

In the following scenario, a surveyor at a large, urban medical center traces the organization's processes and procedures regarding infant and pediatric security. Within the tracer, the surveyor explores issues relating to these priority focus areas:

- Communication
- Orientation and Training
- Patient Safety
- Physical Environment

Scenario

A large, urban medical center is having its triennial survey with a full team in place. At the beginning of the Environment of Care (EC) session, one surveyor notes that the organization has expressed concern about infant and pediatric security in the minutes of its safety committee meetings. When the surveyor speaks with her fellow surveyors at the end of the first day, they comment that staff throughout the organization have also expressed concern about this topic. These concerns prompt the surveyor to trace infant and pediatric security.

(Bracketed numbers correlate to Sample Tracer Questions on page 39.)

➡ **In the Obstetrics Unit.** The surveyor begins the tracer in the obstetrics (OB) unit, first walking around the unit and examining the security systems already in place. Despite the fact that the unit has a state-of-the-art electronic system for controlling access, the surveyor is able to enter the unit unnoticed after a cleared visitor holds the door open for her. Once inside, the surveyor also notes that there is an elevator in the center of the unit that does not seem to be secured.

The surveyor introduces herself to the nurse manager of the unit. She asks if the unit has done a risk assessment for infant abduction and, if so, what the results of that assessment were. [1–2] She also asks what the nurse manager feels the security risks are in the unit and what interventions are in place to address those risks. [3–5]

"I noticed that you have an electronic security system," says the surveyor. "What are the manual processes for security if the electronic security system fails?" "Every staff member on the unit has designated exits he or she must monitor during an electronic security system failure," says the nurse manager. "We monitor who enters the unit and make sure that they have proper identification. We also monitor who exits the unit to make sure they are not carrying out anything suspicious." [6–8]

After this exchange, the surveyor mentions that she entered the unit without having to show identification and offers suggestions on how to prevent such breaches in security from happening in the future. She also suggests that the organization work on securing the elevator in the unit, in order to prevent a potential abductor from entering the unit unnoticed.

➡ *Talking to the OB Nurse.* After speaking with the manager, the surveyor approaches a nurse and asks her what the process is for responding to a missing infant. The surveyor specifically probes for information about how the nurse would know that a child is missing, what the nurse herself would do to respond to the incident, and what her peers would do. The surveyor continues the conversation by asking about orientation and training, seeking to discover whether the nurse has received training on this subject and how often it occurs. [12–15]

"Has this organization ever done an infant abduction drill?" asks the surveyor. [16] "Yes, I think it's been about a year or so since they had one," says the nurse. "I'm new here, so I wasn't around for that, but some of my colleagues have talked about it. The organization had an individual pose as someone abducting a patient, and he tried to take a doll out of the unit. One of the nurses at the desk stopped the individual and sounded the Code Pink. It was interesting to hear about. I hope we have an opportunity to do that type of drill again soon."

➡ *In the Pediatrics Department.* After leaving the OB department, the surveyor stops on the pediatrics floor. She seeks out the nurse manager for the area and asks how the department ensures pediatric security. [1–5] She specifically

MOCK TRACER TIP

In addition to the examining previously mentioned locations, it may be helpful when tracing infant and pediatric security to talk to staff in units located by building exits. Even if these units do not treat infants and children per se, because of their proximity to the buildings' exits, staff members in these units should know and be able to describe their roles in securing the exits during a Code Pink situation.

probes for information about how the unit identifies potentially disruptive family situations—such as estrangement or a custody battle. Because most abductions involving children center around a custody issue, the surveyor wants to ascertain how the unit handles these situations—specifically how the unit releases children to noncustodial parents. [9–11]

The surveyor also notes that the pediatrics department does not have controlled access. She asks the manager why this is the case and whether the manager feels that this puts patients at risk. She also discusses ways the unit can preserve the safety of its patients.

The surveyor then stops a technician working on the unit and asks what he knows about pediatric security. She tries to determine whether the employee knows his role and the roles of his peers in responding to a pediatric abduction. She asks about education and training as well as opportunities to practice what he's learned. [12–15]

→ *In the Emergency Department.* After leaving the pediatrics department, the surveyor visits the emergency department (ED) to see what security systems are in place there to prevent infant and pediatric abduction. She notes that there is no electronic monitoring system present; however, when she tries to access the patient care area, a security officer stops her and asks to see identification. She takes a minute to talk with the security officer, asking about his role in ensuring infant and pediatric safety. [17–21]

She then seeks out the manager of the ED and asks a few more questions about security, orientation and training, and responding to an abduction event.

"So, what does the ED do in the event of a Code Pink?" asks the surveyor. "Well," says the ED manager, "we have specific assigned duties that we all follow, including locking down the ED." The surveyor further chats with the manager about those specific duties and how the unit locks down. [22–25]

→ *At the Security Office.* A final stop in the tracer is the security office. The surveyor asks to see the organization's risk assessment for infant and pediatric security and discusses the results of that assessment. [26–28] She also chats with the director of security about the alarm system in the OB unit.

"Is the security system in the OB unit on emergency backup power?" asks the surveyor. "Yes, absolutely!" says the security director. "During a power failure, the system automatically

shifts over to backup power. We also use manual systems during this time—where we monitor the exits and check identification of people entering and exiting the area—to serve as a double backup." [29–30]

The surveyor also asks the security director about recent infant abduction drills, seeking information on what the organization learned from the drills and how those issues are being addressed. [31–36] She then inquires about drills involving other settings besides OB.

→ *Moving Forward.* Based on the tracer, the surveyor might follow up with a discussion on the fact that although the organization has recently done a drill involving abduction from the OB department, it has never done an abduction drill from the ED or the pediatric unit. Although abduction drills are not mandatory, should the organization choose to do another one, it might focus the drill on the ED or the pediatric unit.

At-a-glance
Compliance Strategies

When considering the risks of infant and pediatric abduction, organizations must also consider risks in ambulatory care settings, such as physicians' offices. For example, when a parent brings a sick child to a physician's office along with his or her well children, the organization must think about how it will preserve the safety of the children who are not being seen by the physician. One possible way is to have the parent bring all the children to the exam room and use a privacy curtain in the room to separate well children from the sick child being examined. This prevents the well children from remaining in the waiting room unsupervised.

Scenario 2-1.
Sample Tracer Questions

The bracketed numbers before each question correlate to questions, observations, and data review described in the sample tracer for Scenario 2-1. You can use the tracer worksheet form in Appendix B to develop a mock tracer (*see* an example of a completed tracer worksheet at the end of this section). The information gained by conducting a mock tracer can help to highlight a good practice and/or determine issues that may require further follow-up.

Nurse Manager

[1] Has the organization conducted a risk assessment on infant/pediatric abduction?

[2] What were the results of this risk assessment?

[3] What are your concerns about infant/pediatric security in this area?

[4] How does the organization control access to this area?

[5] How does the organization preserve security for infants and pediatric patients in this area?

[6] What do you do when the electronic system for controlling access fails?

[7] Does the unit have manual systems in place for controlling access?

[8] How does the unit ensure the security of the elevator?

[9] How does the unit identify potentially disruptive family situations—such as estrangement or a custody battle?

[10] How does the unit increase security around a child involved in such situations?

[11] What processes does the organization have in place for releasing a child to a noncustodial parent?

Nurse/Technician

[12] How do you know if an infant/pediatric patient has been abducted?

[13] What is your responsibility when a Code Pink is called?

[14] What is the responsibility of your peers when a Code Pink is called?

[15] How do you notify internal security about an abduction?

[16] Has the organization ever done an infant/pediatric abduction drill?

Security Officer (ED)

[17] What is your role in preserving the security of infants and pediatric patients in the ED?

[18] How do you respond if a child is missing?

[19] Who do you notify if a child is missing?

[20] How does the organization lock down the ED?

[21] How does the organization notify external security?

ED Manager

[22] How does the ED preserve the safety of infants and pediatric patients?

[23] How do you determine if a child is missing?

[24] What do you do if a child is missing?

[25] How much training does the organization provide ED staff about infant security and abduction response?

Director of Security

[26] Has the organization conducted a risk assessment on infant/pediatric abduction?

[27] What were the results of this risk assessment?

[28] What has been done to address concerns about the potential abduction of an infant or pediatric patient?

[29] Is the security system for OB connected to emergency power?

[30] Why do the ED and pediatric unit not have an electronic system for controlling access?

[31] When was the last abduction drill conducted?

[32] Has the organization done abduction drills for pediatric patients?

[33] Has the organization involved outside law enforcement in those drills?

[34] Has the organization done abduction drills for areas outside the OB unit?

[35] What deficiencies did the organization identify in those drills?

[36] How has the organization responded to those drills?

SCENARIO 2-2. Pharmaceutical Security

Summary

In the following scenario, a surveyor traces an organization's processes for ensuring pharmaceutical security. Within the tracer, the surveyor explores issues relating to these priority focus areas:

- Communication
- Equipment Use
- Medication Management
- Orientation and Training
- Physical Environment

Scenario

While tracing the care of a patient, a surveyor notices a few medication distribution cabinets that are unlocked and unsecured. This prompts him to trace pharmaceutical security throughout the organization.

(Bracketed numbers correlate to Sample Tracer Questions on pages 41–42.)

➡ *On a Patient Care Unit.* The surveyor starts the tracer by speaking with the nurse who dispenses medication to the patient the surveyor is currently tracing. He asks her how she accesses medications to give to patients. She indicates that the unit has both dispensing cabinets and a medication closet. The surveyor asks the nurse whether the dispensing cabinets are regularly locked and how someone can access those cabinets. [1–4] He tries to determine whether staff must use a key to unlock the cabinets and, if so, where that key is stored and who has access to it. He points out that several of the cabinets are unlocked and asks the nurse why she thinks this might be the case. [5] He is trying to identify whether there any "workarounds," (*see the* Mock Tracer Tip on page 41) going on that could present an opportunity for medical error.

The surveyor then talks with another nurse on the unit, asking her if she knows how to ensure the security of medications distributed on the unit.

"Have you received any orientation or training on medication security?" the surveyor queries. "Well, if we have, it's not been much," says the nurse. "I know that the cabinets should remain locked, but I'm not sure why that's so important. It's kind of a pain to keep track of that key and constantly have to lock and unlock the cabinet." [6–7] The surveyor takes a moment to

reinforce the importance of keeping the cabinets locked.

Next, the surveyor approaches the nurse manager for the unit and asks her to show him the medication closet. Together, they verify that the closet is locked, and the nurse manager shows the surveyor where the key is and how that closet can be accessed. He asks about training for staff on medication security and how often that training occurs. He also queries the manager about how the unit prevents drug diversion (that is, removing drugs for illicit use). [8–16] Finally, the surveyor asks whether the organization has done any proactive risk assessments on the topic of medication security. Because he observed some unlocked medication carts, he thinks that performing a risk assessment might be valuable. [17] Also, some further training for staff on the importance of keeping things locked would be beneficial.

The surveyor walks through a couple more patient care units in addition to the one previously mentioned. Throughout all of these units, he notices that the medication cabinets are not always secured appropriately, reinforcing his thought that performing a risk assessment might be valuable.

At-a-glance

Compliance Strategies

As described previously, assessing risks associated with medication security can be beneficial for an organization. The following are some factors to consider within such a risk assessment:

- The number and severity of security incidents within the pharmacy or other units distributing medications
- The level of access to an area or a department that houses medications
- The security hardware present in an area that houses medications, including monitored alarm systems, automatic door locks, and closed-circuit video surveillance systems
- The degree of public traffic through the area as well as the degree of isolation
- The potential degree of loss associated with a security incident, such as the theft of narcotics or other illicit drugs
- Community risks
- The security risks associated with particular times of day

➡️ *At the Pharmacy.* After he looks through the units, the surveyor visits the pharmacy. He notes that the area has controlled access, and he is required to show identification before being allowed to enter. He meets the pharmacy director and asks him to describe the security measures in place in the pharmacy, including who can access the pharmacy and how they do that. [18–20]

He also asks about how the pharmacy prevents diversion of medications. He reviews the pharmaceutical inventory and discusses how the pharmacy staff create the inventory, how often it's reviewed, and what the response would be to missing medications. [21–24] He also probes for information about potentially high-risk medications.

"Do you store narcotics here?" asks the surveyor. "Yes," responds the pharmacy manager. "Over here in this locked cabinet. Only one other pharmacist who works the night shift and I have the key to this storage area. We have to document any time narcotics are removed, how much is removed, and for what purpose. This documentation has to be confirmed by another individual, to make sure no one is removing narcotics on his or her own." [25–27] As with the unit manager, the surveyor discusses the need for a possible risk assessment for medication security with the pharmacy manager. [28]

➡️ *At the Security Office.* A final stop in the tracer is the security office. The surveyor asks the director of security if the organization has had any security incidents related to medication security—specifically medication diversion. He asks about what is involved in responding to an incident and how often incidents are reviewed. [29–32]

➡️ *Moving Forward.* Based on the tracer, the surveyor might follow up with a discussion on conducting a multidisciplinary risk assessment of medication security in the organization. The risk assessment might include individuals such as direct care staff, nurse managers, the pharmacy manager, pharmaceutical staff, and security personnel on the assessment team—as well as a senior leader, as this issue has the potential to negatively affect the organization and its patients. [33]

Scenario 2-2.
Sample Tracer Questions

The bracketed numbers before each question correlate to questions, observations, and data review described in the sample tracer for Scenario 2-2. You can use the tracer worksheet form in Appendix B to develop a mock tracer (see an example of a completed tracer worksheet at the end of this section). The information gained by conducting a mock tracer can help to highlight a good practice and/or determine issues that may require further follow-up.

Nurse on the Unit
[1] How do you access medications to give to patients?
[2] How are those medications kept secure?
[3] Are the cabinets kept locked?
[4] Who has access to those cabinets?
[5] I have noticed that some cabinets are unlocked. Why do you think that is?
[6] Have you received any orientation or training on medication security?
[7] How often do you receive this training?

Nurse Manager
[8] Is the medication closet locked at all times?
[9] Who is allowed access to that closet?
[10] How can you prevent unauthorized access?
[11] How can authorized personnel access the cabinet?
[12] What training does the unit provide on medication security?
[13] How often is this training provided?

(continued)

MOCK TRACER TIP

Medication security can be ripe for workarounds. A *workaround* is a shortcut that a staff person might take to save time. For example, if an employee is leaving the medication storage closet for a short time and is afraid of getting "locked out" of the area because of an automatic latching door, he or she may disable a door latch to ensure that the door remains open. Although this and other types of workarounds may save time for the employee in the short term, such workarounds can present significant safety and security hazards. During the mock tracer process, organizations should be looking for workarounds and identifying ways to eliminate them.

[14] How does the organization prevent medication diversion?

[15] Has the organization ever experienced a diversion event?

[16] How do you respond to such an event?

[17] Has the organization considered doing a risk assessment on medication security?

Pharmacy Manager

[18] Describe the security measures in place in the pharmacy.

[19] Who can access the pharmacy?

[20] How does the organization prevent unauthorized access?

[21] What are the organization's processes for preventing diversion?

[22] How does the organization create the medication inventory?

[23] How often is that inventory reviewed?

[24] How do you respond when medication is missing?

[25] Show where the organization stores narcotics and other high-risk medications.

[26] How does the organization prevent unauthorized access to these medications?

[27] How often are the logs associated with these medications reviewed?

[28] Has the organization ever considered doing a risk assessment on medication security?

Security Officer

[29] Has the organization ever had an incident involving medication security? If so, describe it.

[30] What processes are in place to respond to a medication security incident, such as diversion?

[31] How does the organization notify the proper authorities?

[32] Have security personnel received training and orientation on medication security?

[33] Has the organization ever done a risk assessment on medication security?

SCENARIO 2-3. Security of Radioactive Material

Summary

In the following scenario, a surveyor at a big-city medical center conducts a tracer that examines the security of radioactive isotopes entering the hospital. Within the tracer, the surveyor explores issues relating to these priority focus areas:

- Communication
- Orientation and Training
- Patient Safety
- Physical Environment

Scenario

A surveyor is tracing the care of a patient who has kidney disease and requires a series of diagnostic tests in the radiology department, using nuclear medicine. As part of the tracer, the surveyor visits the radiology department to talk with staff members there about how they conduct nuclear medicine tests for the patient. During this discussion, the topic of securing the radioisotopes used in the nuclear medicine equipment comes up. The surveyor decides to explore this security issue further.

(Bracketed numbers correlate to Sample Tracer Questions on page 44.)

➡️ ***In the Radiology Hot Lab.*** The surveyor goes to the organization's radiology hot lab, located in the building's basement, where the organization stores its radioisotope supply. The hot lab serves several purposes, including storing fresh isotopes and holding spent product while it decays (to make transport easier during removal). The surveyor is accompanied by the radiology manager and asks about the process for deliveries, including how the organization receives isotopes. The surveyor focuses on how the isotopes come in to the organization, are transported through the organization, and end up at the hot lab. [1–4]

"What is your process for receiving radioisotopes?" asks the surveyor. "We have a very specific protocol that governs this effort," says the radiology manager. "We use a licensed and bonded courier who is contracted by the radio pharmacy that creates the isotopes to deliver them. When he or she arrives at the hospital, the courier checks in with the security department and shows identification. The security department calls radiology, and we send someone up to meet the courier. This individual walks the courier to the hot lab, following a very specific path. Once here, we check the courier in to the hot lab and again look at his or her identification. This is, of course, what happens when isotopes are delivered during the day. For night delivery, the whole process goes through the security department. You may want to ask them how they handle that."

The surveyor proceeds to ask more questions about maintaining the security of the isotopes, including where the isotopes are stored and how the hot lab maintains security around that storage area. [5–7] He also asks how radioisotopes are sent to the radiology department for use in nuclear medicine equipment and how the organization ensures safety and security during this transport process. [10]

➡️ *Asking About Cobalt-60 and Emergency Drills.* The surveyor asks the radiology manager whether the organization stores cobalt-60—a radioactive material used in some medical equipment, which has a very long half life and thus could be useful in making dirty bombs. The manager acknowledges that the organization does house some of this material and discusses the specific security precautions around it, including how its delivery and storage processes differ from those of other radioactive material. [8–9]

Finally, the surveyor seeks information on any emergency management (EM) drills the organization has conducted that relate to the security of radioisotopes. According to the radiology manager, the organization has not done such a drill. The surveyor recommends evaluating this topic as part of the organization's hazard vulnerability analysis (HVA; *see* Section 8). He also suggests putting this topic on the organization's list of possible drills because the hospital is located in an urban area with a high-density population and there is a risk that someone could remove the cobalt-60 or other material for use in a terrorist event. [17]

➡️ *Back at the Radiology Department.* After visiting the hot lab, the surveyor makes a brief stop back at the radiology department to meet with a radiology technician who operates the nuclear medicine equipment. The surveyor asks her to show him how radioisotopes are used in the equipment and to discuss how she maintains safety and security of these isotopes. He also asks whether the employee is aware of the health risks associated with the isotopes and any precautions she should take to preserve her safety and that of the patient. He queries her about training and orientation regarding radioisotopes and how often that occurs. [10–15]

➡️ *At the Security Department.* As a final stop, the surveyor visits the security department, where he asks a security officer on duty how he would respond to a delivery of

---

At-a-glance

Compliance Strategies

Only a licensed and bonded courier should deliver radioisotopes to a health care organization. This courier must follow hospital policy regarding facility entrance and travel to the hot lab. Hospital policy may involve providing the courier with key or key card access to the hot lab or requiring the courier to check in with security. In the latter case, security personnel may escort the courier to the hot lab. Regardless of what approach an organization chooses, it must document this protocol and ensure that practice follows policy.

MOCK TRACER TIP

It may be helpful when tracing the security of radioisotopes to actually walk the path a courier would travel when delivering the material. This can allow the organization to see any risks that may not be apparent in just talking with staff in the radiology and security departments.

---

radioisotopes. The employee outlines the same process as the radiology manager.

"What if the delivery arrives in the middle of the night and there are not radiology personnel on site?" asks the surveyor. "Oh, we have a protocol for that as well," says the security officer. "The courier checks in with security, and the security person on duty escorts the courier to the hot lab and waits inside the hot lab until the courier has stored the material. I have to add, though, that before I would leave the security station to accompany the courier, I would make sure that another security officer remains in the security department while I'm away." [16]

➡️ *Moving Forward.* Based on the tracer, the surveyor might follow up with a discussion on including the topic of radioisotope safety in the organization's next EM exercise. Although the processes the organization has in place seem quite effective, testing the processes could be beneficial for the organization. [17–18]

Scenario 2-3.
Sample Tracer Questions

The bracketed numbers before each question correlate to questions, observations, and data review described in the sample tracer for Scenario 2-3. You can use the tracer worksheet form in Appendix B to develop a mock tracer (*see* an example of a completed tracer worksheet at the end of this section). The information gained by conducting a mock tracer can help to highlight a good practice and/or determine issues that may require further follow-up.

Radiology Manager

[1] How does the organization receive radioisotopes?

[2] How are radioisotopes transported through the organization?

[3] How does the hot lab receive radioisotopes?

[4] How does the hot lab maintain the security of radioisotopes during transportation?

[5] Where are the radioisotopes stored in the hot lab?

[6] Who has access to that storage area?

[7] How does the hot lab maintain the security of that storage area?

[8] Does the organization use cobalt-60?

[9] How does the organization maintain the security of this radioactive material?

Radiology Department Employee

[10] How are radioisotopes transported to the radiology department?

[11] How are radioisotopes used in the nuclear medicine equipment?

[12] What are the safety and security risks associated with radioisotopes?

[13] What personal protective equipment should you wear when interacting with radioisotopes?

[14] What protection do patients require?

[15] Have you been trained on how to use radioisotopes properly?

[16] How does the organization receive after-hours delivery of radioisotopes?

Security Officer

[17] Has the organization conducted an emergency drill related to this topic?

[18] What were the results of that drill?

SCENARIO 2-4. Security of the Helistop

Summary

In the following scenario, a surveyor at a Level I trauma center conducts a tracer addressing the security of the organization's helistop. Within the tracer, the surveyor explores issues relating to these priority focus areas:

- Communication
- Equipment Use
- Orientation and Training
- Patient Safety
- Physical Environment
- Staffing

Scenario

One her first day surveying a Level I trauma center, a surveyor notes that the organization has a helistop for transporting critical patients into and out of the facility. Curious about how the organization maintains security and ensures safety regarding the helistop, the surveyor decides to trace the issue.

(Bracketed numbers correlate to Sample Tracer Questions on page 46.)

➡ *At the Facility Manager's Office.* To begin the tracer, the surveyor asks the facility manager to show her the organization's license for operating the helistop as well as the other regulatory paperwork regarding the helistop. [1–3] She asks the facility manager how long the helistop has been in place and what the maintenance requirements are for this location. [4–5] She also asks about fire safety for this location and what type of fire equipment is required. [6–9]

Next, the surveyor asks whether the hospital has a list of companies that are licensed to land at the helistop. "What kind of relationship do you have with these companies?" asks the surveyor. "We stay in touch with them pretty frequently," responds the facility manager. "We have all their contact information on file, and once a year we ask a representative from each company to come on site for a brief meeting about the helistop. At this meeting, we go over any new information about the helistop, including revised security procedures, infection control issues, fire safety issues, maintenance issues, and so on. This helps us communicate with the companies using the helistop, but it also gives them an opportunity to tell us about any issues they are having with our facility or processes. During the rest of the year, we tend to communicate via phone and e-mail." [10–11]

➡ *At the Security Manager's Office.* When she finishes her conversation with the facility manager, the surveyor moves on to the security manager. She asks him what the security issues are with the helistop and how the organization addresses those issues. [12] Specifically, she asks whether the organization has done a risk assessment regarding the helistop to identify all the various trouble spots associated with the area. [13–14]

The surveyor then queries the security manager about specific security issues. "So, how do you limit access to the helistop?" asks the surveyor. "We use a card access system that limits access to only designated hospital helicopter staff and security," says the security manager." We just installed the system about eight months ago, and it has significantly reduced the likelihood that anyone who is not supposed to be in the helistop area could create an unsafe condition on the landing pad. Flight dispatchers can grant access to the helistop for plant operations personnel and others through a combination of cameras and an intercom." [15]

The surveyor and the security manager then discuss other ways the organization ensures the security of the helistop area, focusing on how the hospital keeps the area well lit and secure even when no one is using it. [16] After further discussion about training and orientation for the helistop, the surveyor asks to see the area. The security manager takes her up to the roof, where the surveyor observes how the security processes work in the area and notes any safety issues, including loose wires, debris, and tripping hazards.

➡ *In the ED.* After visiting the helistop, the surveyor goes to the ED, where she speaks with a nurse on duty. She asks the nurse how he knows when a helicopter is approaching the helistop with a critical patient. The nurse mentions the radios that the ED uses to communicate with the different helicopter companies and shows the surveyor where those radios are kept. They discuss how the clinical staff communicate with the people aboard the helicopter to determine what state the patient is in and how to prepare for treatment. [17–18]

"Once you know a patient is on his or her way, how would you access the helistop?" asks the surveyor. "We have a dedicated elevator that provides direct access to the helistop," says the nurse. "We use a special key to call the elevator, and it takes us to the helistop floor and directly back to the ED." The nurse shows the surveyor where the key is stored and talks about who has access to it. [19–20]

MOCK TRACER TIP

To further examine the safety and security risks associated with a helistop, an organization may want to include the use of the helistop in its next EM drill. Helicopters can be an important resource for evacuating people from a hospital, and the organization should consider testing how the helistop will be used in case of emergency.

At-a-glance
Compliance Strategies

An organization should know who has regulatory authority over its helistop and what the local, state, and federal requirements are. It needs to obtain helicopter and helistop information regularly from the relevant agencies to stay up to date with safety, security, construction, and maintenance regulations. Some important sources to consult include the following:

- *The Federal Aviation Administration (FAA).* The FAA's most recent *Helistop Design Guide* (#150-5390-2B), released September 20, 2004, is a good resource.
- *The Centers for Disease Control and Prevention (CDC).* The CDC provides guidelines for infection control practices in helicopters.
- *The National Fire Protection Association (NFPA).* NFPA 419 provides information on constructing and maintaining a helistop.
- *International fire and building codes.* These codes provide fire protection and prevention regulations for helistops.

Finally, the surveyor asks about any training and orientation the nurse has had about how to safely approach a helicopter on the landing pad and what to do in case of emergency, such as a fire. [21] They talk about special equipment used to extinguish fires on the helistop, and the nurse refers the surveyor to the facilities department for more information on that topic.

→ *Moving Forward.* As the surveyor is finishing her tracer, a call comes in about a patient approaching in a helicopter. The surveyor is given the opportunity to watch how staff access the helistop, retrieve the patient from the helicopter, bring the patient to the ED, and begin treatment. This allows the surveyor to fully understand the organization's processes. Based on this review, the surveyor might follow up with a discussion on someone in the department taking notes about an actual helistop response, so the organization can determine whether there are any areas for possible improvement.

Scenario 2-4.
Sample Tracer Questions

The bracketed numbers before each question correlate to questions, observations, and data review described in the sample tracer for Scenario 2-4. You can use the tracer worksheet form in Appendix B to develop a mock tracer (*see* an example of a completed tracer worksheet at the end of this section). The information gained by conducting a mock tracer can help to highlight a good practice and/or determine issues that may require further follow-up.

Facility Manager

[1]   What regulations must the organization follow for its helistop?

[2]   What paperwork is required for the helistop?

[3]   Where is that paperwork stored?

[4]   How does the organization maintain the safety of the helistop?

[5]   What maintenance issues are associated with the helistop?

[6]   How does the organization ensure fire safety of the helistop?

[7]   What equipment is required?

[8]   Who is designated to use that equipment?

[9]   What training does the organization provide staff on that equipment?

[10]   Does the organization have a list of companies that use the helistop?

[11]   What is the organization's relationship with these companies?

Security Manager

[12]   What are the security issues associated with the helistop?

[13]   Has the organization ever done a risk assessment on the helistop?

[14]   What were the results of this assessment?

[15]   How does the organization control access to the helistop?

[16]   How does the organization maintain security even when no one is present at the helistop?

ED Nurse

[17]   How do you know when a helicopter is approaching the helistop?

[18]   How do you communicate with individuals on the helicopter?

[19]   How do you access the helistop?

[20]   Who is allowed to access the helistop?

[21]   What training have you received on the helistop?

Sample Tracer Worksheet: Scenario 2-3.

The worksheet below is an example of how organizations can use the sample tracer questions for Scenario 2-3 in a worksheet format during a mock tracer. The bracketed numbers before each question correlate to questions described in the scenario.

A **correct answer** is an appropriate answer that meets the requirements of the organization and other governing bodies. An **incorrect answer** should always include recommendations for follow-up.

Tracer Team Member(s): Daniel Craigson
Subjects Interviewed: Jack Adams, Yemen Kelmatis, David Bernwell
Tracer Topic: Security of radioactive material

Data Record(s): logs of sign-in and security check
Unit(s) or Department(s): Radiology hot lab, radiology department, security office

Interview Subject: Radiology Manager

Questions	Correct Answer	Incorrect Answer	Follow-Up Needed	Comments or Notes
[1–3] How does the organization receive radioisotopes? How are radioisotopes transported through the organization? How does the hot lab receive radioisotopes?	✓			Describes specific process for receiving isotopes—including use of licensed and bonded courier. Also describes who from the hot lab goes to meet the isotopes and escort them through the building.
[4] How does the hot lab maintain the security of radioisotopes during transportation?		✓	Need to work with staff and empower them with other ways to maintain security of isotopes during transportation.	Aside from escorting the isotopes through the building, the staff member cannot describe other ways to maintain security.
[5–7] Where are radioisotopes stored in the hot lab, who has access, and how does the hot lab maintain security there?	✓			Shows me the storage area and describes ways that security is maintained in that area. The area has key card access, and only the radiology manager and one other staff member have a key. The security department also has a key, should that be necessary.

(continued)

Interview Subject: Radiology Manager (continued)				
Questions	**Correct Answer**	**Incorrect Answer**	**Follow-Up Needed**	**Comments or Notes**
[8–9] Does the organization use cobalt-60? If so, how does the organization maintain the security of this radioactive material?		✓	Need to brainstorm ways to preserve security when cobalt-60 is in transit from the supplier to the machine. Once in the machine, the material is secure, but security is lax during transport.	Yes, there is cobalt-60. It is stored in the machine it's used in, and that machine is locked at all times. Only the radiology manager and the security department have access to the part of the machine that houses the cobalt-60. One weakness: Organization does not have processes in place for maintaining security when cobalt-60 is placed in the machine.

Interview Subject: Radiology Department Employee				
Questions	**Correct Answer**	**Incorrect Answer**	**Follow-Up Needed**	**Comments or Notes**
[10] How are radioisotopes transported to the department?	✓			Comprehensively describes how radioisotopes arrive in the unit and the security measures in place during transport. Radiology manager accompanies all radioisotopes to the unit and oversees installation.
[11–15] How are radioisotopes used in the nuclear medicine equipment, and what safety precautions are needed with this effort, and have you been properly trained?		✓	Should conduct another tracer on employee safety with regard to radioactive material. Initial thoughts from this tracer show that further education is needed for staff members on how to ensure their own and the patient's safety.	Can describe how radio isotopes are used but is a little sketchy on the risks involved in using them. Describes the personal protective equipment adequately but cannot articulate how to preserve the patient's safety and why that is important. This topic may warrant another tracer to further explore employee safety during radioactive material use.

Interview Subject: *Security Officer*				
Questions	**Correct Answer**	**Incorrect Answer**	**Follow-Up Needed**	**Comments or Notes**
[16] How does the organization receive after-hours delivery of radioisotopes?	✓			Adequately describes the process for receiving an after-hours delivery of radioisotopes. Training on this issue seems to be sufficient.
[17–18] Has the organization conducted an emergency drill on this topic? What were the results?		✓	Consider performing a drill on this topic or incorporating it into the next EM exercise that relates to terrorism.	No drill as of this time. Suggest one in the future to plug potential holes in the system.

Tracer Scenarios for
HAZARDOUS MATERIALS AND WASTE

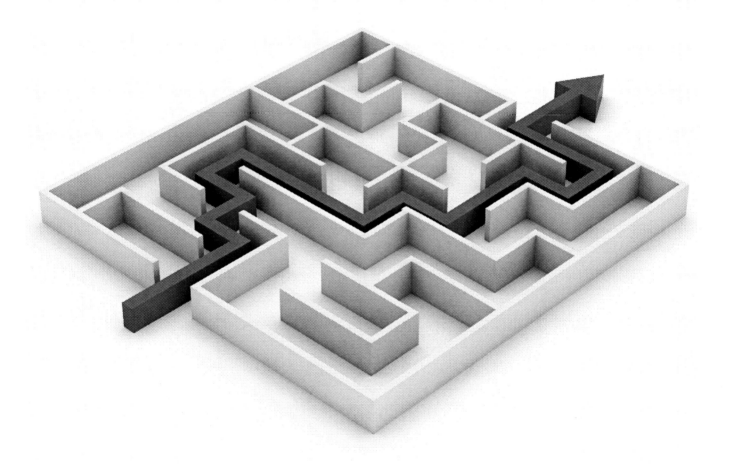

NOTE: No Two Tracers Are the Same

Please keep in mind that each tracer is unique. There is no way to know all of the questions that might be asked or documents that might be reviewed during a tracer—or what all the responses to the questions and documents might be. The possibilities are limitless, depending on the tracer topic and the organization's circumstances. These tracer scenarios and sample questions are provided as educational or training tools for organization staff; they are not scripts for real or mock tracers.

Section Elements

This section includes sample tracers—called scenarios—relevant to hazardous materials and waste. The section is organized as follows:

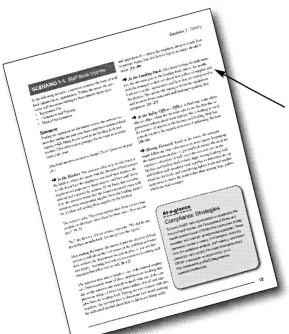

Scenarios: Each scenario presents what might happen when a surveyor conducts a specific type of tracer. The scenarios are presented in an engaging narrative format in which the reader "follows" the surveyor through the tracer scenario. Within the narrative are bracketed numbers that correspond to numbered sample tracer questions following the tracer.

Sample Tracer Questions: After each scenario narrative is a list of sample questions a surveyor might ask during that scenario. These questions can be used to develop and conduct mock tracers in your organization on topics similar to those covered in the scenario.

Sample Tracer Worksheet: At the end of the section is a sample worksheet that shows how the sample tracer questions for one select scenario in the section might be used in a worksheet format. The example shows how the worksheet might be completed as part of a tracer for that scenario. A blank form of the worksheet is available in Appendix B.

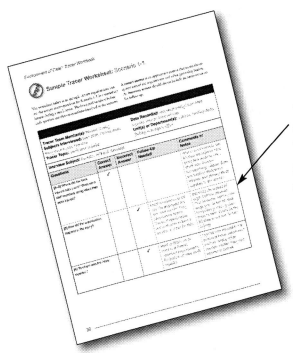

SCENARIO 3-1. Laboratory Safety

Summary

In the following scenario, a surveyor conducts a tracer that closely examines the environmental conditions in an organization's laboratory, specifically focusing on how the laboratory handles and disposes of hazardous materials and waste. Within the tracer, the surveyor explores issues relating to these priority focus areas:

- Equipment Use
- Orientation and Training
- Physical Environment

Scenario

As a surveyor reviews the minutes of an organization's Environment of Care (EC) committee, he notices that there have been two hazardous materials spills in the laboratory in the past 18 months. This serves as a red flag to the surveyor and prompts his decision to pay a visit to the laboratory to investigate how it manages its hazardous materials and waste.

(Bracketed numbers correlate to Sample Tracer Questions on pages 54–55.)

➡️ *At the Office of the Safety Officer.* Before visiting the laboratory, the surveyor stops by the office of the safety officer and asks for all the data the organization has on hazardous materials spills in the laboratory. He asks how these data are compiled and how often the safety officer reviews the information. [1–3] He engages in a brief conversation with the safety officer about whether he thinks the incidents represent a pattern in laboratory safety. [4]

"Is the laboratory part of your environmental tours process?" asks the surveyor. [5] "Of course," says the safety officer. "We visit it at least once a year, and that's documented on the form we use during the process." "Can I please see the form?" requests the surveyor.

The safety manager produces the form. As the surveyor reviews it, he notices that there are several issues not present on the form that probably should be. For example, the form does not reflect activities such as looking at expiration dates for hazardous materials, examining overcrowding issues, or verifying staff members' comfort level with spill response. After reviewing the form, the surveyor asks the safety officer to accompany him to the laboratory.

➡️ *At the Laboratory.* Upon entering the laboratory, the surveyor notes that the room is crowded and has several potential safety hazards for tripping, spilling, and so forth. He further examines the area by opening cupboards, checking behind doors, and looking in several other places to get a sense of how the laboratory stores its hazardous materials. He makes note of any flammable materials and checks to see if they are stored appropriately. During this brief examination, he discovers one material that, according to the label, is expired.

"How do you check to see if your hazardous materials are expired?" asks the surveyor. [6] "We have a list of hazardous materials that are here in the lab, and the list includes the expiration dates for the different materials—along with other things, like the chemical name of the materials, the personal protective equipment (PPE) required when handling the materials, the storage location, and the health and fire risks associated with the materials," says the laboratory manager. "Once every six months, I review the list to make sure we don't have any hazardous materials that have expired." The surveyor points out the expired material to the laboratory manager and suggests that he consider reviewing the list more frequently.

The surveyor then asks how the laboratory labels and stores its hazardous materials, focusing specifically on how it stores flammable materials and those with look-alike and sound-alike names. He checks whether the labels follow regulatory requirements, including those of the Occupational Safety and Health Administration, The Joint Commission, and the National Fire Protection Association. He asks the manager if there are any other regulatory bodies that govern the laboratory's processes for labeling and storing hazardous materials. [7–11]

MOCK TRACER TIP

When tracing hazardous materials, it can be helpful to spend some time reviewing the organizationwide chemical inventory. The EC standards require organizations to create and maintain such a chemical inventory and consider criteria consistent with applicable law and regulation when developing it. Although the Scenario 3-1 mentions part of the inventory that is housed in the laboratory, an organization should also have an organizationwide inventory that lists all the hazardous chemicals found across the facility.

The surveyor then asks how the laboratory disposes of any expired hazardous material or waste. He probes for information on where the material is sent for disposal, how it gets there, and how the laboratory ensures its safety en route. He also discusses what methods of disposal are available at the organization. [12–13]

The surveyor points out that the laboratory is very crowded and presses the laboratory manager about why this is so. The laboratory manager expresses his frustration with the amount of materials the laboratory is required to store and indicates that the space is not sufficient to do so adequately. [14]

➡ *Talking with a Lab Technician.* After speaking with the laboratory manager, the surveyor approaches a laboratory technician and asks her if he can speak with her about her work with hazardous materials. During this conversation, the surveyor asks the technician what hazardous materials she works with, what risks are associated with the material, what PPE she uses, how much training and education she's had on the material, and what she does if she spills some of the material. [15–19]

"Could you show me the material safety data sheet (MSDS) for this material?" asks the surveyor. "Sure, it's kept on the computer here, and I can bring it up online for you," says the technician. After watching the technician access the electronic MSDS, the surveyor asks about what plans the organization has in place should the power go out or the Internet go down. The laboratory technician is not sure what to do in those situations and suggests that the surveyor ask her manager. [20–21]

At-a-glance
Compliance Strategies

To ensure that hazardous materials and waste are treated appropriately, an organization should consider maintaining a reference library of all applicable federal, state, and local laws and regulations. Maintenance of this library helps demonstrate that all the various regulatory requirements have been considered. If an organization is unable to refer to the actual regulations, it is difficult to see what requirements the hazardous materials and waste program is based on and how the organization keeps abreast of changes to applicable regulations.

The surveyor follows up with the manager and finds out that the laboratory does have a binder that houses all MSDSs in the lab. He suggests that the laboratory manager provide more training to his staff about how and when to access that binder.

➡ *Moving Forward.* Based on the tracer, the surveyor might follow up with a discussion on these topics: the laboratory manager and the safety officer collaborating to update the EC tours form to reflect more accurately all the possible safety issues associated with the laboratory; the laboratory manager reviewing how the lab is laid out and where items are stored to minimize the crowding issue and ensure that the environment is safe for staff; how leadership might help the laboratory manager address the problem of the laboratory crowding; and the need for sufficient staff training regarding hazardous materials.

Scenario 3-1.
Sample Tracer Questions

The bracketed numbers before each question correlate to questions, observations, and data review described in the example tracer for Scenario 3-1. You can use the tracer worksheet form in Appendix B to develop a mock tracer (*see* an example of a completed tracer worksheet at the end of this section). The information gained by conducting a mock tracer can help to highlight a good practice and/or determine issues that may require further follow-up.

Safety Officer

[1] How does the organization collect data on hazardous materials and waste spills?

[2] Are these data available for specific locations, such as the laboratory?

[3] How often do you review these data?

[4] Do you think the incidents in the laboratory represent a pattern of risk?

[5] Is the laboratory part of the environmental tours process?

Laboratory Manager

[6] How do you check to see if your hazardous materials are expired?

[7] How does the laboratory label its hazardous materials?

[8] How does the laboratory store its hazardous materials?

[9] How does the laboratory store its flammable materials?

[10] How does the laboratory store materials with look-alike and sound-alike names?

[11] What regulatory bodies control the laboratory's storage, labeling, and handling of hazardous materials and waste?

[12] How does the laboratory dispose of any expired material or waste?

[13] Describe the who, what, where, and when of the disposal process.

[14] Why is the laboratory so crowded?

Laboratory Technician

[15] What hazardous materials do you work with?

[16] What risks are associated with the hazardous materials?

[17] What PPE do you use?

[18] What training and education have you had on these materials?

[19] What would you do if you spilled some of these materials?

[20] How do you access the MSDS for this material?

[21] How do you access an MSDS when the computer is not available?

SCENARIO 3-2. Responding to a Spill

Summary

In the following scenario, a surveyor traces how an organization responds to a hazardous materials and waste (hazmat) spill. Within the tracer, the surveyor explores issues relating to these priority focus areas:

- Communication
- Orientation and Training
- Patient Safety
- Physical Environment

Scenario

A surveyor who is part of a three-member survey team is chatting with her fellow surveyor at the end of the first day. During this conversation, the other surveyor mentions that he spent 30 minutes tracing the organization's processes for managing hazardous materials and waste in the laboratory. He notes that the staff member in the laboratory with whom he spoke was familiar with how to respond to a hazmat spill, but the surveyor is curious about whether staff in other depart-

ments, such as housekeeping and staff on patient care units, would be as knowledgeable on this issue. The first surveyor offers to trace this topic on her next survey day.

(Bracketed numbers correlate to Sample Tracer Questions on pages 56–57.)

➡️ ***On a Patient Care Unit.*** The surveyor starts her tracer on a patient care unit that houses some hazardous materials. She asks a nurse's assistant what hazardous materials the unit has. [1] Although there aren't very many, the assistant does list a few, including liquid nitrogen. The surveyor asks the nurse's assistant to describe what would happen if someone spilled liquid nitrogen on the floor. [2] During this conversation, the surveyor asks about how the spill would be initially cleaned and disinfected; what PPE would be necessary when cleaning up the spill; how and when staff, patients, and leadership would be notified of the spill; when to evacuate the area; how to respond to exposed individuals; and how to prevent exposure to others in the organization, such as patients and staff outside the spill area. [3–8] The surveyor realizes that the staff member may not be able to articulate all the details in the response, but she is looking to discover whether the staff member understands what her role is in the response and who she should notify if the spill is beyond her ability to address.

"Let's say this is a really large spill," says the surveyor. "Who would you call to address that?" "We have a hazmat response team," responds the nurse's assistant. "I would call them to our unit over our intercom system using the 'hazmat one' code and our unit number." [9]

The surveyor completes her conversation with the nurse's assistant by asking her about training and education she's received on spill response. They discuss a recent online training that included

MOCK TRACER TIP

When conducting a mock tracer on how to respond to a hazardous materials spill, an organization may want to retrace the steps in its last actual hazmat spill response. If possible, someone should talk to the people who discovered the spill, cleaned up the spill, notified the fire department, and so forth. This will allow the organization to see how it truly would respond to a hazmat incident.

this topic and some posters in the unit that describe the proper response. [10]

➡ *At the Housekeeping Department.* After speaking to the nurse's assistant, the surveyor stops by the housekeeping department and talks with the manager on duty. She asks what the housekeeping department's role is in cleaning up spills—specifically those related to hazardous cleaning materials, such as bleach. [11] As with the nurse's assistant, the surveyor probes for details about the spill response, including who a housekeeping staff member would call should a spill surpass his or her abilities to respond appropriately. [2–8]

➡ *At the Facility Manager's Office.* Finally, the surveyor stops by the facility manager's office to find out who the members of the hazmat response team are. She asks to speak to one of these individuals and is immediately introduced to a senior

maintenance person, who leads the team. She asks him who is on the team, how they are trained, and what their response to a spill would be. [12–14]

"When do you notify outside authorities, such as the fire department?" asks the surveyor. [15–16] "Our local fire department has a hazmat unit, and they will come on site here whenever we have a large spill," responds the maintenance person. "The job of our internal hazmat spill team is just to contain the spill and then to contact the fire department. We have met with the fire department to talk about how this works, and they have walked through our facility, so they know what areas are most likely to have a large hazmat spill. We have also worked with them to develop procedures for responding to a spill to make sure our efforts complement theirs."

➡ *Moving Forward.* The surveyor asks the maintenance person if the organization has ever done a spill response drill specifically focusing on a spill in which someone needs decontamination. [17–18] The maintenance person says that the organization is considering such a drill. The surveyor strongly suggests pursuing this idea and involving the local fire department and other emergency responders in the drill.

At-a-glance
Compliance Strategies

Training and education are key to effective hazmat spill response. Depending on the nature and scope of a spill, a staff member may or may not have a lot of involvement in cleaning it up. For this reason, organizations should consider providing different levels of training, depending on the individual's role in the spill response. For example, within the basic training, organizations could train staff members to do the following:

- Clean up a spill of hazardous material only if they have the training and equipment to do so.
- Alert others in the area of the chemical spill.
- If possible, keep the area ventilated.
- If possible, try to contain the spill with absorbent materials until the spill responders arrive.
- If possible, get a copy of the MSDS to assist the responder.
- If possible, turn off all ignition and heat sources.
- Contact appropriate personnel in the event of a large-scale spill.

More advanced training could address all these topics plus how to clean up specific types of spills and when to contact the fire department.

Scenario 3-2.
Sample Tracer Questions

The bracketed numbers before each question correlate to questions, observations, and data review described in the example tracer for Scenario 3-2. You can use the tracer worksheet form in Appendix B to develop a mock tracer (*see* an example of a completed tracer worksheet at the end of this section). The information gained by conducting a mock tracer can help to highlight a good practice and/or determine issues that may require further follow-up.

Nurse's Assistant

[1] What hazardous materials does this the unit have?

[2] What would happen if someone spilled one of these hazardous materials?

[3] How would the spill be cleaned and disinfected?

[4] What PPE would be necessary when cleaning up the spill?

[5] How would you notify other staff, patients, and leadership about the spill?

[6] When would you need to evacuate the area?

[7] How would you respond to exposed individuals?

[8] How would you prevent exposure to others in the organization?

[9] Who would you call to address a really large spill?

[10] What training and education have you received on spill response?

Housekeeping Manager

[11] What is the housekeeping department's role in cleaning up spills, specifically those related to hazardous cleaning materials such as bleach?

Head of the Hazmat Response Team

[12] Who is on the hazmat response team?

[13] How are these team members trained?

[14] What is the team's response to a hazmat spill?

[15] When do you notify outside authorities, such as the fire department?

[16] What is the organization's relationship with the fire department regarding hazmat response?

[17] Has the organization ever done a spill response drill?

[18] Has such a drill included an individual who needs decontamination?

SCENARIO 3-3. Infectious Waste Disposal

Summary

In the following scenario, a surveyor traces an organization's processes for infectious waste disposal. Within the tracer, the surveyor explores issues relating to these priority focus areas:

- Infection Control
- Orientation and Training
- Patient Safety
- Physical Environment

Scenario

During the initial day of patient care tracers, a surveyor notices several staff members improperly handling infectious waste on patient care units. For example, he observes certain staff members dragging waste bags across the floor, placing discarded needles and other sharp instruments (commonly called "sharps") in unapproved containers, and leaving waste bags unattended. These observations prompt the surveyor to trace infectious waste disposal throughout the organization.

(Bracketed numbers correlate to Sample Tracer Questions on pages 58–59.)

→ *On a Patient Care Unit.* The surveyor first approaches a nurse on a patient care unit who has just discarded a syringe into the trash. "I notice that you threw that in the trash," says the surveyor. "Is that the proper way to dispose of a used syringe?" [1] "I think so," says the nurse. "This is how we all do it. I know we have those red plastic containers for sharps, but I thought those were only for syringes used with infectious patients. This person is healthy, so I thought I could just throw it in the regular trash."

The surveyor spends some time with the nurse, further asking her about how she disposes of other infectious waste, such as bloody gauzes or soiled paper table covers. He tries to discover whether the nurse is aware of the risks associated with this infectious waste and what the proper ways are to dispose of it in order to protect herself and others. During this time, he further probes for information about training and education on infectious waste disposal. [2–6]

He then speaks with the supervisor on the unit, who is able to describe the organization's policy regarding used syringe disposal. The surveyor points out that there may be a training issue here, because he is noting several staff members who are seemingly not aware of the organization's policy and are disposing of syringes improperly. [7–8]

→ *At the Elevator.* After leaving the unit, the surveyor notices a housekeeping staff person waiting by the elevator holding a red bag of infectious waste. He approaches the staff person and asks her some questions about the material she's holding, including from where she retrieved the bag and what types of materials are in the bag. [9–10]

MOCK TRACER TIP

The standards governing the disposal of infectious waste are now found in the "Infection Prevention and Control" chapter. So, when doing a mock tracer, organizations should involve both EC and infection control (IC) professionals in the effort as both play an active role in ensuring the proper disposal of these materials. Infection preventionists and EC professionals should work together to create and implement a coordinated approach to tracing the waste stream.

"What PPE do you wear when you handle this type of bag?" asks the surveyor. **[11]** "I always wear gloves like these," says the housekeeping staff person, as she points to the pair of gloves she's wearing. "There is a box of these next to each one of the red bag containers, so I usually just grab a pair from there."

The surveyor follows up this exchange with a query about how the staff person ensures that the elevator buttons don't become contaminated because the staff person is using the same gloves while handling the bag. **[12]** He also asks her about any training and education she has received about infectious waste disposal. **[13]** When describing her training, the staff person comments that it would be nice if the organization could provide training in both English and Spanish because many of her coworkers don't speak English well.

The surveyor then asks the housekeeping staff person to walk him through the process of retrieving a red bag infectious waste container, transporting it through the organization, and bringing it to the loading dock for removal from the building. During this tour, he notes several times when infection control (IC) is compromised and clean items come in contact with the infectious waste bag.

➡ *At the Loading Dock.* At the loading dock, the surveyor speaks with the loading dock manager to determine how the infectious waste is stored until the contracted infectious waste hauler arrives for pickup. He probes for details about the hauler, including how the organization selected this particular contractor. He also asks the loading dock manager how he documents the arrival and removal of infectious waste. **[14–18]**

At-a-glance
Compliance Strategies

Infectious waste must be handled in a manner that minimizes the hazard to the handler, other staff, patients, and visitors. Organizations should consider the travel paths of infectious waste and sterile or clean supplies within the building so that the two do not come into regular contact. Infectious waste processing areas should be separated from "clean" areas. Organizations should also ensure that an appropriate holding area is provided for materials that are shipped off site for disposal.

➡ *At the IC Department.* A final stop is the IC department, where the surveyor speaks with the manager there. He probes for information about the organization's policies on infectious waste disposal, including who develops those policies, how they are maintained, and what training is provided to staff on those policies. **[19–22]**

➡ *Moving Forward.* Based on the tracer, the surveyor might follow up with a discussion on improving training and education for staff.

Scenario 3-3.
Sample Tracer Questions

The bracketed numbers before each question correlate to questions, observations, and data review described in the example tracer for Scenario 3-3. You can use the tracer worksheet form in Appendix B to develop a mock tracer (*see* an example of a completed tracer worksheet at the end of this section). The information gained by conducting a mock tracer can help to highlight a good practice and/or determine issues that may require further follow-up.

Nurse on a Patient Care Unit

[1] What is the proper way to discard of a used syringe?

[2] How do you discard soiled gauzes or other infectious waste?

[3] What are the risks associated with infectious waste?

[4] What PPE should you wear when handling infectious waste?

[5] What training and education have you had about infectious waste disposal?

[6] How often does that training occur?

Supervisor on a Patient Care Unit

[7] What training does the organization provide on infectious waste?

[8] How does the organization measure whether that training is effective?

Housekeeping Staff Member

[9] From where did you retrieve that bag?

[10] What types of materials are in that bag?

[11] What PPE do you wear when you handle this type of bag?

[12] How do you ensure IC when transporting the bag?

[13] What training and education have you received on infectious waste disposal?

Loading Dock Manager

[14] How does the organization store infectious waste at the dock until the contracted infectious waste hauler arrives for pickup?

[15] Who is the organization's hauling contractor?

[16] How did the organization choose that contractor?

[17] How do you document when infectious waste arrives on the loading dock?

[18] How do you document when the contractor picks up the infectious waste?

IC Manager

[19] What are the organization's policies on infectious waste disposal?

[20] Who develops these policies?

[21] How often are these policies reviewed?

[22] What training does the organization provide to staff on these policies?

SCENARIO 3-4. Radiation Safety

Summary

In the following scenario, a surveyor explores the issue of radiation safety in an organization. Within the tracer, the surveyor explores issues relating to these priority focus areas:

- Orientation and Training
- Patient Safety
- Physical Environment

Scenario

A surveyor is tracing the care of a patient who requires radiation therapy. Aware of the serious health and safety risks associated with providing radiation therapy, the surveyor decides to explore the ways the organization maintains the safety of staff and patients who interact with radiation.

(Bracketed numbers correlate to Sample Tracer Questions on pages 60–61.)

➡ *In the Nuclear Medicine Preparation Area.* The surveyor first visits with a physicist in the nuclear medicine prepa-

ration area. They discuss how the physicist prepares radioactive source material and how he minimizes exposure risk. [1–3] Specifically, the two focus on what technology the physicist uses to prevent exposure. [4] The surveyor asks about PPE, including lead aprons and other shielding devices. [5] He also asks the physicist to describe how he would respond to and report an exposure to radiation. [6–7]

"What training have you had regarding the safe preparation of radioactive source material?" asks the surveyor. [8] "They train us quite frequently about this topic because it's so important," responds the physicist. "I received an initial orientation when I started two years ago, and the hospital offers refresher courses online every six months. The online course also has some downloadable material that I print out and take home to read later. My department also has posters hanging up in the area that describe what to do in case of an exposure to radiation and who to call."

After speaking with the physicist, the surveyor spends some time observing the preparation area, noting how staff members interact with, prepare, and dispose of radioactive material. He also looks for personal exposure dosimeter badges on staff who work with radiation and verifies that none of the badges appear to be showing dangerously high levels of radiation. He stops a staff members wearing one of these badges and asks why she is wearing the badge and how to interpret it. He is trying to establish that the staff member is familiar with how to respond to dangerous readings. [9–10]

➡ *On a Patient Care Unit.* After leaving the nuclear medicine preparation area, the surveyor stops by a patient care unit that performs radiation therapy. He approaches a physician who is working on the unit and asks to speak with her about radiation therapy. During this conversation, the surveyor and the physician talk about the process for handling radioactive source material, from delivery through administration and then disposal. [11] They discuss PPE involved in handling the material as well as what training and education the physician has received on safe practices regarding radiation. [12–13]

➡ *Interviewing a Patient.* The surveyor approaches a patient receiving radiation therapy. "What education have you received regarding your treatment and safety precautions?" asks the surveyor. [14] "I have to say, the hospital has been pretty thorough about educating me," says the patient. "Before I started my treatment, I talked it over with the physician and nurse, and they also sent me home with a video about radiation therapy. It explained the risks involved in such therapy and how the organization was going to protect me as much as possible from those risks. They also gave me some written information, but I couldn't get through it. It was way too difficult. My daughter, who is in medical school, had a hard time understanding it!"

The surveyor then asks the patient what staff members wear when giving her the radiation treatment and asks her to describe how the treatment is administered. With this conversation, the surveyor is trying to determine whether the organization's practices regarding radiation therapy match its procedures. [15–16]

➡️ *In the Housekeeping Department.* After visiting the patient care unit, the surveyor stops by the housekeeping department, where he speaks with one of the housekeeping staff

members who cleans the patient care units that engage in radiation therapy. During this conversation, he focuses on how the staff member removes the radioactive material from the unit and disposes of it. They discuss PPE as well as her use of a personal dosimeter exposure badge. He probes for how the staff member reports an exposure to radiation and to whom. Finally, they discuss training and orientation. [17–23]

After chatting with the housekeeping staff member, the surveyor asks if he can follow her for a bit because he wants to see how she handles and disposes of the radioactive waste. Specially, he wants to see how the housekeeping staff member transports the radioactive waste to its final disposal area. He also wants to monitor her dosimeter badge.

➡️ *Moving Forward.* As a last stop, the surveyor visits the safety officer to see if the organization has done a risk assessment on radiation safety. [24–25] The safety officer indicates that the organization did do one, but it's been a few years. Based on this, the surveyor might follow up with a discussion on revisiting the exercise and looking at how the organization can enhance education for both patients and staff, including staff in preparation areas, on patient care units, and within the housekeeping department.

At-a-glance
Compliance Strategies

Radiation dosimeter badges are helpful tools for measuring staff members' exposure to radiation in real time. Often battery operated, these audible detectors are worn on a staff member's clothing and measure the amount of alpha, beta, gamma, and x-radiation present. Staff should know how to respond to readings showing an increased exposure level. Such response may include removing themselves from the situation and seeking medical treatment. If an organization uses dosimeter badges, it must make sure staff members are appropriately trained on the importance of the badges and how to read them. Otherwise, staff may eventually work around or ignore the badges.

MOCK TRACER TIP

As part of a mock tracer on radiation safety, an organization may want to ask staff members who prepare radioactive materials to demonstrate how they don and doff PPE, where they access such PPE, and what they do with it once it's been used. Appropriate use of PPE is critical when handling these dangerous materials.

Scenario 3-4.
Sample Tracer Questions

The bracketed numbers before each question correlate to questions, observations, and data review described in the example tracer for Scenario 3-4. You can use the tracer worksheet form in Appendix B to develop a mock tracer (*see* an example of a completed tracer worksheet at the end of this section). The information gained by conducting a mock tracer can help to highlight a good practice and/or determine issues that may require further follow-up.

Physicist in the Nuclear Medicine Preparation Area

[1] How do you prepare radioactive source material?

[2] What risks are involved in preparing such material?

[3] How do you minimize the risk of exposure?

[4] What technology do you use to prevent exposure?

[5] What PPE do you wear when preparing radioactive source material?

[6] Describe how you would respond to an exposure to radiation.

[7] To whom would you report such an exposure?

[8] What training have you had regarding the safe preparation of radioactive source material?

[9] Why are you wearing that badge?

[10] How do you interpret the information on the badge?

Physician

[11] What is the process for handling radioactive source material, from delivery through administration and then disposal?

[12] What PPE do you use when handling radioactive material?

[13] What training and education have you received on safe practices with regards to radiation?

Patient

[14] What education have you received regarding your radiation treatment and safety precautions?

[15] What do staff members wear when giving you radiation treatment?

[16] Describe, as best you can, how radiation treatment is administered.

Housekeeping Personnel

[17] How do you remove radioactive material from the unit?

[18] How do you dispose of such material?

[19] What PPE do you wear when removing radioactive material from the unit?

[20] How does the dosimeter badge work?

[21] How do you report exposure to radiation?

[22] To whom do you report such exposure?

[23] What training and education have you received about radioactive material handling?

The Safety Officer

[24] Has the organization done a risk assessment on radiation safety?

[25] If so, what were the results of that assessment?

Sample Tracer Worksheet: Scenario 3-3.

The worksheet below is an example of how organizations can use the sample tracer questions for Scenario 3-3 in a worksheet format during a mock tracer. The bracketed numbers before each question correlate to questions described in the scenario.

A **correct answer** is an appropriate answer that meets the requirements of the organization and other governing bodies. An **incorrect answer** should always include recommendations for follow-up.

Tracer Team Member(s): James May
Subjects Interviewed: Yolanda Vargas, Irene Stiffler, Mary Rodriguez, Jack Mayweather, Betsy Morgan

Tracer Topic: Infectious waste disposal
Data Record(s): haz mat logs; DOT logs/manifests
Unit(s) or Department(s): Patient care unit, housekeeping department, loading dock, infection control

Interview Subject: Nurse on a Patient Care Unit

Questions	Correct Answer	Incorrect Answer	Follow-Up Needed	Comments or Notes
[1] What is the proper way to discard a used syringe?		✓	Need training for staff on proper syringe disposal.	Staff suggest throwing syringes in regular trash, not hard-sided red plastic containers. This presents both infection control and injury hazards.
[2] How do you discard soiled gauzes or other infectious waste?	✓		Should reinforce this in training efforts.	Knew to throw soiled materials in infectious waste container.
[3] What are the risks associated with infectious waste?		✓	Need comprehensive and regular training on this topic.	Could not articulate all the risks involved in handling infectious waste. Specifically unaware of risks involving sharp needles. Also not fully aware of risks associated with bloodborne pathogens.
[4] What PPE should you wear when handling infectious waste?	✓			Is able to show the appropriate PPE for handling infectious waste. Indicates the use of gloves and sometimes double gloves.

Interview Subject: Nurse on a Patient Care Unit (continued)				
Questions	**Correct Answer**	**Incorrect Answer**	**Follow-Up Needed**	**Comments or Notes**
[5–6] What training and education have you had about infectious waste disposal? How often does that training occur?		✓	Need to closely examine training and orientation for this topic. Suggest offering different types of training—online tutorials, posters, in-services, etc. May want to involve IC department in developing these.	Received initial training during orientation 5 years ago. Can't remember any refresher training. Didn't observe any posters or signage about infectious waste disposal.

Interview Subject: Supervisor on a Patient Care Unit				
Questions	**Correct Answer**	**Incorrect Answer**	**Follow-Up Needed**	**Comments or Notes**
[7–8] What training does the organization provide on infectious waste? How does the organization measure the success of this training?		✓	Work with IC department to revamp training and ensure that the success of training is measured. This topic needs to be more of a priority for the organization. Should involve leadership in this topic and training efforts.	Confirms comment by nurse—not much training on this topic and no tests of success. Not sure this is a priority for the organ

Interview Subject: Housekeeping Staff Member				
Questions	**Correct Answer**	**Incorrect Answer**	**Follow-Up Needed**	**Comments or Notes**
[9–10] From where did you retrieve that bag? What types of materials are in that bag?	✓			Staff member able to clearly describe where she got the bag and what types of material are in it.
[11] What PPE do you wear when you handle this type of bag?		✓	Review processes for transporting infectious waste and ensure that policy matches practice. Also provide training for housekeeping staff about how frequently to change gloves.	Although staff member describes PPE well, she indicates that she uses the same gloves over and over when transporting red bags instead of changing gloves.

(continued)

Interview Subject: Housekeeping Staff Member (continued)

Questions	Correct Answer	Incorrect Answer	Follow-Up Needed	Comments or Notes
[12–13] How do you ensure IC when transporting the bag? What training and education have you received on infectious waste disposal?		✓	IC and EC need to work together to trace the path of infectious waste and develop procedures to ensure that waste does not present IC issues. Training should be offered on these revised procedures.	Could not demonstrate IC procedures while transporting bag.

Interview Subject: Loading Dock Manager

Questions	Correct Answer	Incorrect Answer	Follow-Up Needed	Comments or Notes
[14] How does the organization store infectious waste at the dock until the contracted infectious waste hauler arrives for pickup?	✓			Able to show locations where infectious waste is stored. This location seems appropriate and safe, with minimal IC risks.
[15–16] Who is the organization's hauling contractor? How did the organization choose that contractor?	✓		May want to review selection criteria for the contractor since contract review is coming up in 6 months. Should involve both IC and EC staff in developing these criteria.	Able to identify contractor and describe systematic process for selection. Manager indicates that they review the contract every 3 years. Hauling contractor is up for review in 6 months.
[17] How do you document when infectious waste arrives on the loading dock?		✓	Create a process for documenting infectious waste arrival. This might include the name of the person bringing the waste into the department, the number of bags of waste, the arrival time, etc.	Could not describe a process for documenting infectious waste's arrival at the loading dock.

Interview Subject: Loading Dock Manager (continued)				
Questions	**Correct Answer**	**Incorrect Answer**	**Follow-Up Needed**	**Comments or Notes**
[18] How do you document when the contractor picks up the infectious waste?	✓		Create a system for matching "bags in" to "bags out." This prevents losing bags of waste. Loading dock manager, IC manager, and EC manager should work on this process.	Do have form that contractor signs when picking up infectious waste. This form shows the number of bags and the time of removal. Although this is good, there is no system for ensuring that the number of bags of waste coming onto the loading dock matches the number of bags leaving the loading dock. Need to create this process.

Interview Subject: IC Manager				
Questions	**Correct Answer**	**Incorrect Answer**	**Follow-Up Needed**	**Comments or Notes**
[19–22] What are the organization's policies on infectious waste disposal? Who develops these policies? How often are they reviewed? What training does the organization provide to staff on these policies?	✓		Need to do a comprehensive review of the policies. Should involve walking the waste stream. As mentioned before, need to do a comprehensive overhaul on training for this topic. Should train staff at all levels, test retention after training, and retrain often. Also, should create posters and clever reminders—perhaps a mnemonic on how to dispose of infectious waste.	Is able to show written policies for infectious waste disposal. Were developed by IC staff several years ago. Have not been reviewed in more than a year. Training offered during orientation but not in regular staff training.

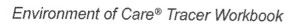

Tracer Scenarios for
FIRE SAFETY

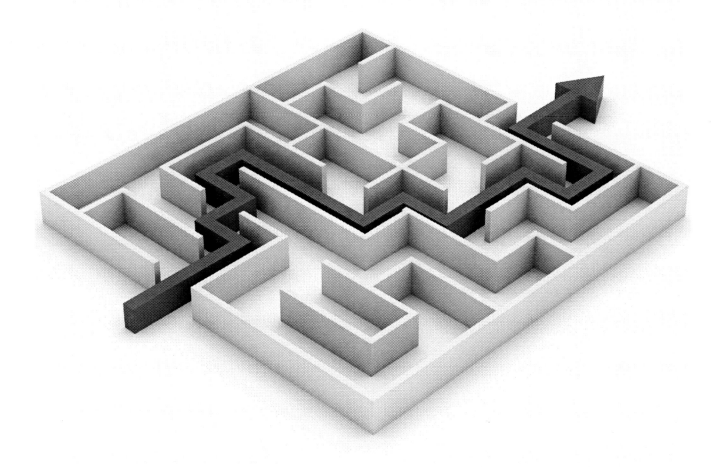

NOTE: No Two Tracers Are the Same

Please keep in mind that each tracer is unique. There is no way to know all of the questions that might be asked or documents that might be reviewed during a tracer—or what all the responses to the questions and documents might be. The possibilities are limitless, depending on the tracer topic and the organization's circumstances. These tracer scenarios and sample questions are provided as educational or training tools for organization staff; they are not scripts for real or mock tracers.

Section Elements

This section includes sample tracers—called scenarios—relevant to fire safety. The section is organized as follows:

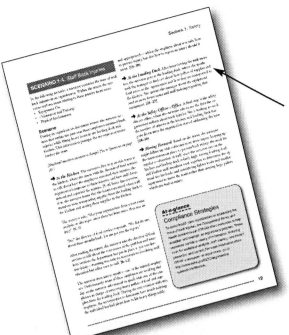

Scenarios: Each scenario presents what might happen when a surveyor conducts a specific type of tracer. The scenarios are presented in an engaging narrative format in which the reader "follows" the surveyor through the tracer scenario. Within the narrative are bracketed numbers that correspond to numbered sample tracer questions following the tracer.

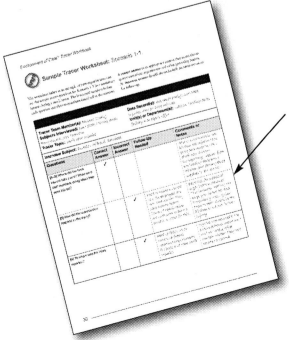

Sample Tracer Questions: After each scenario narrative is a list of sample questions a surveyor might ask during that scenario. These questions can be used to develop and conduct mock tracers in your organization on topics similar to those covered in the scenario.

Sample Tracer Worksheet: At the end of the section is a sample worksheet that shows how the sample tracer questions for one select scenario in the section might be used in a worksheet format. The example shows how the worksheet might be completed as part of a tracer for that scenario. A blank form of the worksheet is available in Appendix B.

SCENARIO 4-1. Fire Plans

In the following scenario, a surveyor traces an organization's fire plan and ensures that practice matches policy. Within the tracer, the surveyor explores issues relating to these priority focus areas:

- Communication
- Orientation and Training
- Patient Safety
- Physical Environment

Scenario

During an organization's Environment of Care (EC) session, a surveyor spends some time reviewing the organization's fire plan. She is curious about whether the staff throughout the organization understand and can articulate the different actions discussed in the plan, and so she decides to trace the topic.

(Bracketed numbers correlate to Sample Tracer Questions on page 70.)

➡ *During the EC Session.* To begin the tracer, the surveyor asks the safety officer, security director, facility manager, and maintenance director a few questions about the fire plan, including how they create and maintain the plan, who is involved in this process, and how often they review the plan. [1–3] She also asks what training organization staff receive on the fire plan and how often staff familiarity with the plan is tested. [4–5] She then asks these leaders to describe a recent fire drill and its outcomes. [6]

Next, the surveyor selects a particular patient unit and asks the EC leaders what the expectations are of staff on the unit when responding to a fire. [7] She follows up by asking to visit the unit under discussion.

➡ *On the Patient Unit.* When the surveyor arrives on the unit, she asks to speak with the unit manager. They discuss the unit's approach to fire response and how often that approach is tested. The surveyor also asks about any training and education the unit has received on the organization's fire response plan. [8–13] Her goal for this conversation is to see if the manager's understanding of fire response mirrors what is written in the plan.

The surveyor then selects a specific staff member with whom to talk. "If there were a fire on this unit in Room 312, what would you do?" asks the surveyor [14]. "It's my job to close all

the doors to patient rooms in the event of a fire, so that's probably what I would do first," says the staff member. "One of my coworkers would pull the alarm and contact the fire response team, and another one would move everything out of the hallway and close the hallway doors."

The surveyor asks what would happen next, including how the staff member would ensure the safety of patients on the unit and when the unit would make the decision to evacuate. They discuss both horizontal and vertical evacuations, with the staff member identifying where the unit would meet as a group in the event of an evacuation. [15–21]

"You mentioned a fire response team," says the surveyor. "Who is on that team?" [22–23] "As far as I know, the team is made up of members of the maintenance and security departments," says the staff member. "In the event of a fire, this team would come to the unit before the fire department arrives and help us contain the fire."

After talking with the staff member, the surveyor stops and talks with the staff member's colleagues about their role in the fire response, checking to see if their answers match those of the original staff member. [14–16] She asks these staff members what their response would be if the fire were on the fourth floor, in the unit above the one they're in. In this conversation, she is trying to determine whether the staff members understand their role both at the location of the fire and away from it as well as their general awareness of fire drills. [25–26]

➡ *In the Maintenance Department.* As a final stop on the tracer, the surveyor goes to the maintenance department and asks to speak with the individual in charge of the fire response team. The surveyor asks him several questions about how the team would be notified of a fire, what their response

MOCK TRACER TIP

Another area of the organization that can be helpful to trace regarding fire response is the operating room. Staff within this area will have specific responsibilities during a fire, and these will often differ from the responsibilities of staff in other locations. Staff in the operating room should be familiar with their fire response responsibilities, and they should also have practiced them when possible by participating in fire drills.

would be, and how they would coordinate with the fire department. She also asks for information on the type of equipment they would use to contain the fire and where they would access that equipment. Finally, the surveyor asks about recent fire drills and what, if anything, the organization learned during those drills. **[27–35]**

➡️ *Moving Forward.* Based on the tracer, the surveyor might follow up with a discussion on focusing on training and education about fire response when the fire is away from the unit. This training could include further drills that address this topic.

Scenario 4-1.
Sample Tracer Questions

The bracketed numbers before each question correlate to questions, observations, and data review described in the sample tracer for Scenario 4-1. You can use the tracer worksheet form in Appendix B to develop a mock tracer (see an example of a completed tracer worksheet at the end of this section). The information gained by conducting a mock tracer can help to highlight a good practice and/or determine issues that may require further follow-up.

EC Leadership

[1] How does the organization create and maintain the fire response plan?

[2] Who is involved in this process?

[3] How often does the organization review the plan?

[4] What training do staff receive on the fire response plan?

[5] How often are staff understanding and familiarity with the plan tested?

[6] Describe a recent fire drill and what the outcomes of that drill were.

[7] What are the expectations of unit staff in responding to a fire?

Patient Unit Manager

[8] What is the unit's approach to fire response?

[9] How often is this approach tested?

[10] What training and education has this unit had on the fire response plan?

[11] How often is that training provided?

[12] Who provides the training?

[13] How does the organization ensure that the training is effective?

Patient Unit Staff Member

[14] If there were a fire on this unit, what would you do?

[15] How would you ensure the safety of patients?

[16] What would you do about items stored in the corridor?

[17] When would the unit make the decision to evacuate?

[18] Who would make that decision?

[19] How would the unit horizontally evacuate?

[20] How would the unit vertically evacuate?

[21] Where would the unit meet up after the evacuation?

[22] Who is on the organization's fire response team?

[23] What is the role of the fire response team in the fire response?

[24] What would your response be if the fire were on a different floor from yours?

[25] When was the last time your unit participated in a fire drill?

[26] How did the fire drill go?

Fire Response Team Leader

[27] How is the fire response team notified about a fire?

[28] What is the role of the fire response team in responding to a fire?

[29] How does the organization interact with the fire department?

[30] What equipment does the fire response team use to help contain a fire?

[31] Where does the team access that equipment?

[32] Describe a recent fire drill in which you participated.

[33] Did the organization involve the fire department in the drill?

[34] What were the results of the drill?

[35] What did the organization learn from the drill?

At-a-glance
Compliance Strategies

Many health care organizations use the "RACE" (Rescue–Alarm–Confine–Extinguish) acronym to teach staff members about their expected response to a fire. Per the acronym, the first step in fire response is to rescue anyone who is in immediate danger, if it is safe to do so. Then the staff member should sound the fire alarm through whatever mechanism is designated in the facility; this may involve using a pull station, calling the operator, or some combination of notifications. Next, all corridor doors should be closed to contain the fire. Finally, depending again on organizational interpretation, a staff member should either use a fire extinguisher to put out an incipient (early-stage) fire, if it is safe to do so, or begin the evacuation process to an area of refuge on the far side of closed smoke-barrier doors.

SCENARIO 4-2. Response to a Real Fire

Summary

In the following scenario, a surveyor traces an organization's response to a real fire. Within the tracer, the surveyor explores issues relating to these priority focus areas:

- Communication
- Orientation and Training
- Patient Safety
- Physical Environment

Scenario

During an organization's EC session, the surveyor learns that the organization recently experienced a small fire in a storage closet near a patient care unit. No one was hurt in the fire, but the organization did have an opportunity to perform a real-life response effort. The surveyor is interested in finding out how that response went and what, if anything, the organization learned from the experience.

(Bracketed numbers correlate to Sample Tracer Questions on pages 72–73.)

➡️ *At the Unit.* First, the surveyor visits the unit where the fire took place. He asks the manager on duty to describe what happened during the incident, including how the fire started, who discovered the fire, what the initial response was, and how the fire was contained and ultimately put out. [1–5]

"Did the response go according to plan?" asks the surveyor. "For the most part, yes," says the manager. "However, because the fire was in a storage closet off the unit, it took us a little while to figure out where the fire was coming from. We smelled smoke, and one of the staff members began looking around for the source of that smoke. Once he saw the smoke pouring out from under the door to the storage area, we were able to call the fire response team and get the fire under control pretty quickly." "Did you have to evacuate?" "In looking back on it, we may not have had to, but there was a piece of equipment near the storage closet that was getting very hot, and we were afraid it would start to arc, so we did a horizontal evacuation just to be sure. We moved everyone down to the end of the hall, on the other side of the smoke doors." [6–7]

The surveyor probes for details about the evacuation. He asks how quickly the evacuation took place as well as how the staff maintained communication with family members and other organization staff during the evacuation. He also asks when patients were allowed back on the unit and how staff got them there. [8–12]

"Did the evacuation go the way you thought it would? asks the surveyor. [13–14] "Yes, the staff knew what to do, and we were able to do a quick huddle before we evacuated to confirm everyone's responsibilities. This served as a reminder of where to go, what to do, and most of all, how to keep patients safe."

After speaking with the manager, the surveyor talks with one of the nurses who was on duty during the fire. He asks about her perspective on the fire response, including how the fire response team responded to the event, when the fire department arrived, and how the unit interacted with the fire department. [15–19] He also presses for her perspective on the evacuation, how patients were brought back to the unit after the fire, and whether there were any difficulties with this process. They discuss how the unit addressed the odor left by the fire and ensured that it did not negatively affect patients and staff. [20–23]

➡️ *Moving Forward.* After speaking to the nurse, the surveyor goes to the maintenance office, where he speaks to the head of the fire response team. He asks the team leader to describe the response and whether it went according to plan. The surveyor also asks what was done to repair the storage closet after the fire and how that effort went. Finally, the surveyor asks if there was anything about the response that should be done differently in the future. [24–28]

"Although the unit called us pretty quickly, there was a delay from the time they smelled smoke to the time they called us," says the team leader. "I am planning to reinforce at the next training that staff should call the response team at the first whiff of smoke and not wait until they see fire."

At-a-glance
Compliance Strategies

As discussed in this tracer scenario and the preceding one, some organizations have first responder teams that are responsible for quickly responding with an extinguisher to the scene of a fire alarm. If an organization has this function, it should describe it in the fire response plan, and the team members should be given additional training, particularly in the use of fire extinguishers. Be careful in naming the team, however—calling it a "fire brigade" invokes additional Occupational Safety and Health Administration (OSHA) training requirements, which will probably be more than a health care organization needs to provide.

MOCK TRACER TIP

Performing a mock tracer on a real event is always helpful. This process allows an organization to see how its staff respond during changing dynamics and pressure-filled situations. It can also help identify weaknesses in organizational systems and processes that may not appear during a regular tracer. Taking some time after an incident has finished to retrace the events leading up to, during, and after the incident will help provide a unique perspective on an organization's standards compliance.

Scenario 4-2.
Sample Tracer Questions

The bracketed numbers before each question correlate to questions, observations, and data review described in the sample tracer for Scenario 4-2. You can use the tracer worksheet form in Appendix B to develop a mock tracer (*see* an example of a completed tracer worksheet at the end of this section). The information gained by conducting a mock tracer can help to highlight a good practice and/or determine issues that may require further follow-up.

Unit Manager

[1]   How did the fire start?

[2]   Who discovered the fire?

[3]   What was the initial response to the fire?

[4]   How did the organization contain the fire?

[5]   How was the fire ultimately extinguished?

[6]   Did the fire response go according to plan?

[7]   Did the unit have to evacuate?

[8]   How quickly did the unit evacuate?

[9]   How did staff maintain communication with family members and other organization staff during the evacuation?

[10] When were patients allowed back on the unit?

[11] How did staff transport patients back to the unit?

[12] How did staff ensure patient safety during transport?

[13] Did the evacuation go the way you thought it would?

[14] What did the organization learn from the event?

Unit Nurse

[15] How did the unit respond to the fire?

[16] Were you pleased with the response?

[17] How did the fire response team respond to the event?

[18] When did the fire department arrive?

[19] How did the organization interact with the fire department?

[20] How did the evacuation go?

[21] Were there any difficulties with this process?

[22] Did the unit smell like smoke after the fire?

[23] How did the organization address the odor?

Fire Response Team Leader

[24] Describe how the response team responded to the fire.

[25] Did the response go according to plan?

[26] What was done to repair the storage closet after the fire?

[27] How did that repair effort go?

[28] Was there anything about the response that should be done differently in the future?

SCENARIO 4-3. Fire Drills

Summary

In the following scenario, a surveyor reviews an ambulatory care organization's processes for conducting fire drills. Within the tracer, the surveyor explores issues relating to these priority focus areas:

- Communication
- Orientation and Training
- Patient Safety
- Physical Environment

Scenario

When reviewing an ambulatory care organization's written fire response plan, a surveyor decides to trace how the organization conducts fire drills. In this tracer, he is looking to see if the organization performs regular drills, analyzes staff performance in those drills, and uses information gleaned from the drills in performance improvement efforts.

(Bracketed numbers correlate to Sample Tracer Questions on page 74.)

➡ *At the Admissions Desk.* The surveyor first visits the admissions section of the ambulatory clinic and asks if he can chat with an admissions clerk on duty about the organization's fire drills.

"When was the last time you participated in a fire drill here?" asks the surveyor. [1] "I think about a month ago," responds the clerk. "We do them at least once a quarter that I'm aware of." "How does the drill work?" asks the surveyor. [2] "They always do them just before or after normal business hours, so we don't need to involve patients," says the clerk. "The facility manager places an orange cone with the word FIRE written on it somewhere in the clinic. The person who discovers that cone is expected to act as if it were a real fire and pull the fire alarm.

When the alarm sounds, we all have specific responsibilities that we need to do, and then we exit all the way out of the building. At least one person goes out each exit to make sure there are no blocked or locked exits."

The surveyor probes for more details about the admission clerk's specific responsibilities during a drill and asks if she feels comfortable with those responsibilities. He also asks about any training and education the clerk has received on this topic. [3–5]

"Are fire drills usually announced beforehand?" asks the surveyor. "Not usually," says the clerk. "Sometimes they let us know so we can prepare, but most of the time they happen unannounced." [6]

➡ *At the Nursing Desk.* After speaking with the admissions clerk, the surveyor talks with one of the nurses at the

At-a-glance
Compliance Strategies

The number of fire drills an organization needs to conduct each year and the frequency with which it must conduct them depend on the organization's setting and occupancy—health care occupancy, ambulatory care occupancy, residential occupancy, or business occupancy. Health care, ambulatory health care, and residential occupancies must conduct one fire drill per shift of operation per quarter. This includes all hospitals, behavioral health care hospitals, and long term care organizations. Freestanding business occupancies, laboratories, and office-based surgery centers need to conduct only one drill annually per shift. Requirements for home care programs vary. In leased or rented facilities, an organization needs to conduct drills only in areas it occupies.

An organization may want to consider using some sort of tickler system as a reminder of when it is time to do a drill and in what area the drill should take place. It is not necessary to have a drill in each area of an organization's building or buildings each year. A rotating schedule can ensure that all staff members in all areas of all buildings have opportunities to participate over time.

clinic. He asks her many of the same questions he asked the clerk, looking to see if the nurse understands her roles and responsibilities during a fire drill. [1–5] He also chats with a physician on duty about her role in a fire drill.

➡ *At the Facility Manager's Office.* The surveyor stops by the facility manager's office because he is the individual in charge of fire safety for the clinic. The surveyor asks the facility manager how drills are conducted in the organization, including whether the fire department is notified ahead of time. [7–8] The surveyor asks to see the organization's documentation on fire drills and spends some time reviewing that documentation. He then queries the facility manager about fire drill evaluations, trying to discover who conducts the evaluations and how they conduct them. He probes for information on what the organization does with the information collected in the evaluations, seeking to see if the organization uses it to improve response during a fire. [9–15]

➡ *Moving Forward.* Based on the tracer, the surveyor might follow up with a discussion on these topics: improving fire drill evaluations; possibly creating a form to help ensure that all evaluations capture necessary information; and using information gleaned from the evaluations to help improve performance in this area.

MOCK TRACER TIP

When tracing fire drills, it can be helpful to see visually how a drill would work. Although it is not appropriate to simulate an entire fire drill during a mock tracer, asking one staff member physically to walk through his or her responsibilities during a fire drill can be beneficial. Following the staff member's footsteps can help the surveyor visualize the process.

Scenario 4-3.
Sample Tracer Questions

The bracketed numbers before each question correlate to questions, observations, and data review described in the sample tracer for Scenario 4-3. You can use the tracer worksheet form in Appendix B to develop a mock tracer (*see* an example of a completed tracer worksheet at the end of this section). The information gained by conducting a mock tracer can help to highlight a good practice and/or determine issues that may require further follow-up.

Admissions Clerk and Nurse

[1]   When was the organization's last fire drill?

[2]   How was the drill started?

[3]   What was your role in the drill?

[4]   Are you comfortable with that role?

[5]   What training and education have you received on fire response?

[6]   Are fire drills usually announced beforehand?

Facility Manager

[7]   How are drills conducted in this organization?

[8]   Does the organization notify the fire department before the drill so it doesn't respond?

[9]   How does the organization evaluate its fire drills?

[10] Who is in charge of evaluating the drills?

[11] What does the organization do with the information gleaned from the evaluations?

[12] Does the organization use the information for performance improvement?

[13] In the last drill, what was something the organization learned?

[14] What corrective actions were taken as a result of the drill?

[15] Who followed through on those corrective actions?

Sample Tracer Worksheet: Scenario 4-2.

The worksheet below is an example of how organizations can use the sample tracer questions for Scenario 4-2 in a worksheet format during a mock tracer. The bracketed numbers before each question correlate to questions described in the scenario.

A **correct answer** is an appropriate answer that meets the requirements of the organization and other governing bodies. An **incorrect answer** should always include recommendations for follow-up.

Tracer Team Member(s): Jamie Severin
Subjects Interviewed: Lauren Darcy, Jodie Szesniak, Marcus Phelps
Tracer Topic: Response to a real fire

Data Record(s): after-action critique of the organization's fire response; after-action report from responder (fire department)
Unit(s) or Department(s): Patient care unit 4C, maintenance department

Interview Subject: Unit Manager

Questions	Correct Answer	Incorrect Answer	Follow-Up Needed	Comments or Notes
[1–6] Describe how you discovered, responded to, and extinguished the fire. Did the response go according to plan?		✓	Need to work on training patient care staff on when exactly to sound the alarm for a fire and why it's important not to wait.	In describing the situation, the manager mentions that the unit waited to sound the alarm until they discovered where the smoke was coming from. They should have pulled the alarm as soon as they smelled smoke. That way, they could have gotten response personnel on site sooner.
[7–8] Did you have to evacuate? How quickly did you evacuate?	✓			Described the evacuation thoroughly. Seemed to go according to plan. Made good decisions and executed well.
[9] How did staff maintain communication with family members and other organization staff during the evacuation?		✓	Need to work with staff to develop ways to maintain communication during an evacuation—especially with family members and other staff.	The unit didn't have many processes for communicating with families. If the incident had been longer, this could have been a problem.

(continued)

Interview Subject: Unit Manager (continued)				
Questions	**Correct Answer**	**Incorrect Answer**	**Follow-Up Needed**	**Comments or Notes**
[10–14] When were patients allowed back on the unit? How did you transfer them back to the unit? How did you ensure safety? Did the evacuation go the way you thought it would, and what did you learn?	✓		Should pursue how this would happen with a longer-term evacuation, or perhaps even a vertical evacuation.	Manager described how the fire department gave the all-clear to return to the unit. Staff escorted patients back appropriately and safely.

Interview Subject: Unit Nurse				
Questions	**Correct Answer**	**Incorrect Answer**	**Follow-Up Needed**	**Comments or Notes**
[15–16, 20–21] Describe the incident, your role in the incident, what went well, and what didn't go well.	✓			Nurse's perception of the event matches the manager's. She thinks the evacuation went smoothly. Able to describe the procedures for evacuation adequately.
[17–19] How did the fire response team respond to the event? When did the fire department arrive? How did the organization interact with the fire department?	✓			Fire response team arrived almost immediately after receiving the call. The fire department was on site within 5 minutes. The nurse was pleased with the rapid response. She thinks the unit manager could have called earlier, though, to alert the team. Nurse didn't have much interaction with the fire department. She left that to the fire response team.
[22–23] Did the unit smell like smoke after the fire? How did the organization address the odor?	✓			The unit did smell pretty bad after the fire. Nurse worked with maintenance personnel to set up plastic sheets to prevent the smell of smoke from spreading. She frequently checked with patients who have breathing issues to make sure they weren't adversely affected by the smell.

Interview Subject: Fire Response Team Leader				
Questions	**Correct Answer**	**Incorrect Answer**	**Follow-Up Needed**	**Comments or Notes**
[24–25, 28] Describe the response to the fire. Did the response go according to plan? Should anything be done differently in the future?		✓	The fire response team leader should incorporate information on when to call the team in the next training session about fire response. The leader should perhaps even use a video or reenactments to reinforce this.	Described the fire response. It appears to have been an efficient and effective response once the team was called. The delay in calling is potentially problematic. It could have resulted in patient harm in certain circumstances.
[26–27] What was done to repair the storage closet after the fire? How did that repair effort go?	✓			The organization hired a contractor to repair the closet and fix the smoke and fire damage.

Environment of Care® Tracer Workbook

Tracer Scenarios for
MEDICAL EQUIPMENT

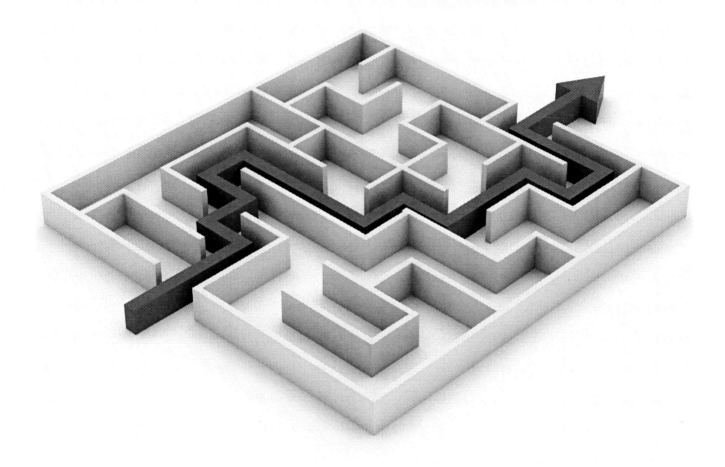

NOTE: **No Two Tracers Are the Same**

Please keep in mind that each tracer is unique. There is no way to know all of the questions that might be asked or documents that might be reviewed during a tracer—or what all the responses to the questions and documents might be. The possibilities are limitless, depending on the tracer topic and the organization's circumstances. These tracer scenarios and sample questions are provided as educational or training tools for organization staff; they are not scripts for real or mock tracers.

Section Elements

This section includes sample tracers—called scenarios—relevant to medical equipment. The section is organized as follows:

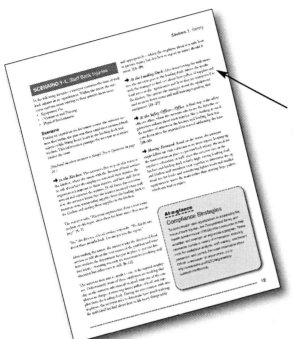

Scenarios: Each scenario presents what might happen when a surveyor conducts a specific type of tracer. The scenarios are presented in an engaging narrative format in which the reader "follows" the surveyor through the tracer scenario. Within the narrative are bracketed numbers that correspond to numbered sample tracer questions following the tracer.

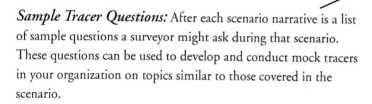

Sample Tracer Questions: After each scenario narrative is a list of sample questions a surveyor might ask during that scenario. These questions can be used to develop and conduct mock tracers in your organization on topics similar to those covered in the scenario.

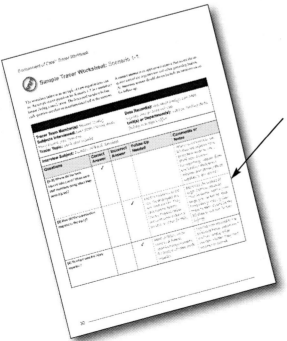

Sample Tracer Worksheet: At the end of the section is a sample worksheet that shows how the sample tracer questions for one select scenario in the section might be used in a worksheet format. The example shows how the worksheet might be completed as part of a tracer for that scenario. A blank form of the worksheet is available in Appendix B.

SCENARIO 5-1. Medical Equipment Maintenance

Summary

In the following scenario, a surveyor traces an organization's system for medical equipment maintenance. Within the tracer, the surveyor explores issues relating to these priority focus areas:

- Communication
- Equipment Use
- Orientation and Training
- Patient Safety

Scenario

At the end of an organization's first full day of survey, two surveyors are chatting about their findings for the day. The first surveyor—a physician—mentions that he noticed during one of his patient care tracers that the radiology department just received some new equipment. The surveyor is curious about the organization's processes for including that equipment on a medical equipment inventory and for ensuring its timely maintenance. The surveyor who is scheduled to conduct the Environment of Care (EC) session the next day says he will follow up on this topic.

(Bracketed numbers correlate to Sample Tracer Questions on page 83.)

➡️ *During the EC Session.* The surveyor first broaches the topic by asking to see the organization's written medical equipment inventory. [1–2] The organization keeps its inventory in a database, and the manager of the biomedical equipment department—who is in charge of creating and maintaining the inventory for this organization—accesses the database for the surveyor to review.

"How do you determine which pieces to include in your inventory?" asks the surveyor, as he peruses the database. [3] "Well, including all medical equipment on the inventory would be unmanageable for us because we have so much medical equipment here," says the biomedical equipment manager. "So, we prioritize and include only those pieces that meet certain risk criteria. These criteria address things like equipment function, physical risks associated with using the equipment, maintenance requirements for the equipment, and equipment incident history. Based on these criteria, we generate a risk-ranking score for each type of equipment and establish a lower cutoff. Anything below the cutoff isn't included on the inventory. Anything above it is. The new equipment we just got for radiology, for example, is certainly on the inventory."

➡️ *Asking About Maintenance.* The surveyor follows up this discussion with questions about how the organization ensures that all equipment listed on the inventory is appropriately maintained. [4–6] The biomedical equipment manager shows the surveyor the section of the database that allows the organization to document maintenance schedules and track maintenance information. He points out that the system can send reminders about maintenance to the individuals in charge of the maintenance activity, which helps ensure that equipment receives maintenance at the appropriate time.

Through this conversation, the surveyor learns that many of the specific maintenance efforts done in the organization occur at the department level. [7] Each department that has responsibility for maintaining equipment has access to the database and updates it when maintenance is done. The biomedical equipment manager also mentions that he holds a medical equipment maintenance meeting every quarter in which the various individuals in charge of maintaining equipment coordinate work and discuss challenges.

After reviewing the minutes of one of the quarterly medical equipment maintenance meetings, the surveyor asks to visit the radiology department to look at its medical equipment and inquire about how the department maintains that equipment.

➡️ *At the Radiology Department.* Upon entering the department, the surveyor introduces himself to the manager and asks her how the various pieces of equipment in the department are maintained, including the various maintenance strategies used for various pieces. He asks about patterns and

MOCK TRACER TIP

When determining where to conduct a mock tracer for medical equipment, it can be helpful to look at the laboratory and radiology departments, since these areas house much of the complex equipment found in a health care organization. In many cases, organizations rely on outside contractors to service laboratory and radiology equipment, so these areas may also present a good opportunity to trace the communication between the organization and any contractors.

trends associated with the equipment and inquires what training is provided to the individuals charged with maintaining the equipment. [9–12] During this conversation, the surveyor learns that some of the equipment is maintained on site and that other pieces are serviced by an outside contractor. The surveyor then reviews the maintenance documentation for the pieces that are maintained on site. He focuses on the records for one particular piece to ensure that there is documentation for the previous 12 months.

The surveyor then presses for information on how designated pieces are sent out to the contractor and what is done with that equipment when it's returned to the unit. The surveyor also asks to see the contract of the maintenance company. [13–18]

"How do you communicate with medical equipment users about equipment maintenance?" asks the surveyor. [19] "We affix a replaceable sticker on each piece of equipment that shows when maintenance was performed, who performed it, and what type of maintenance was done," says the manager. "This allows us to communicate with users about the status and safety of the equipment. The sticker system also allows us to quickly see when a piece of equipment needs to be serviced. The due date for service is also logged in our medical equipment database."

After speaking with the manager, the surveyor walks around the unit and checks all the equipment, looking for stickers and verifying that maintenance was done at the required intervals.

The surveyor then approaches a clinical staff member and asks her about her role in responding to a medical equipment issue. He is checking to see if she is able to explain who to call to report the issue and how to respond to the patient if the equipment fails while it is in use. [20–24]

➡ *Moving Forward.* As a final stop in this tracer, the surveyor goes to the office of the biomedical equipment manager and asks whether the organization has ever used the data in the medical equipment database to track performance. [8] For example, has the organization ever looked at the number of times a particular piece of equipment has failed and worked to address possible underlying issues with that equipment? Has the organization ever rethought maintenance strategies for pieces of equipment that fail often? The biomedical equipment manager indicates that he performs an annual review of the medical equipment database and looks for trends and patterns that might raise concerns. The surveyor discusses how the biomedical equipment manager might continue this effort and work

collaboratively with others tasked with equipment maintenance to address any concerning issues.

At-a-glance
Compliance Strategies

Following is a list of several types of maintenance strategies for medical equipment. An organization might want to consider using a combination of these to develop an effective maintenance program:

- *Interval-based maintenance:* This is the strategy that most health care organizations use. It calls for given pieces of equipment to be maintained on a regular, calendar-based schedule, such as weekly, monthly, or semiannually, regardless of equipment condition.

- *Predictive maintenance:* This strategy is based on an "if–then" algorithm. It allows the adjustment of maintenance cycles based on the presence or absence of a predictor.

- *Reliability-centered maintenance:* This type of maintenance is based on a historical analysis of the reliability of the equipment. The organization then anticipates maintenance activities to extend the reliability based on intersecting historical failure.

- *Metered maintenance:* This type of maintenance is based on the established amount of time the equipment has operated rather than a calendar schedule. It can look at the total run time of the equipment or the number of starts and stops.

- **Run-to-fail maintenance:** This basically involves running the equipment until it malfunctions, at which time the equipment is simply replaced or exchanged with a functioning device.

- *Corrective maintenance:* Sometimes known as user-requested maintenance, this strategy does not service equipment based on preventive models but allows it to run until repairs are needed. When equipment fails, it is assessed, repaired, and returned to service as quickly as possible.

Scenario 5-1.
Sample Tracer Questions

The bracketed numbers before each question correlate to questions, observations, and data review described in the sample tracer for Scenario 5-1. You can use the tracer worksheet form in Appendix B to develop a mock tracer (*see* an example of a completed tracer worksheet at the end of this section). The information gained by conducting a mock tracer can help to highlight a good practice and/or determine issues that may require further follow-up.

Biomedical Equipment Manager

[1] How does the organization create its medical equipment inventory?

[2] How often does the organization review the inventory?

[3] How does the organization determine which pieces to include in its inventory?

[4] How does the organization ensure that all equipment is appropriately maintained?

[5] What various maintenance strategies does the organization use?

[6] How does the organization track maintenance schedules and information?

[7] How do you communicate with various departments in charge of medical equipment maintenance?

[8] Has the organization ever used the data in the medical equipment database to track performance?

Radiology Manager

[9] How does this department maintain various pieces of medical equipment?

[10] What maintenance strategies does the department use?

[11] What patterns have you seen with this equipment?

[12] What training is provided to the individuals charged with maintaining the equipment?

[13] How does the department handle medical equipment that is serviced off site?

[14] Who is the contractor the department uses to maintain the equipment?

[15] How do you communicate with this contractor?

[16] How do you get the equipment to the contractor?

[17] How does the organization ensure that the contractor is doing a good job?

[18] What do you do to ensure that equipment returned to your location is in working order?

[19] How do you communicate with medical equipment users about equipment maintenance?

Clinical Staff

[20] What do you do if a piece of equipment you are using fails?

[21] Who do you call to report this failure?

[22] How do you get the equipment fixed after it fails?

[23] How do you maintain the safety of patients during an equipment failure?

[24] Who do you contact with questions about the equipment?

SCENARIO 5-2. Product Recalls

Summary

In the following scenario, a surveyor examines an organization's processes for responding to product recalls. Within the tracer, the surveyor explores issues relating to these priority focus areas:

- Communication
- Equipment Use
- Patient Safety

Scenario

During a patient care tracer, a surveyor is talking with a physician about a piece of medical equipment used in treatment. As part of the tracer, the surveyor asks the physician about the organization's product recall process, including the process for responding

MOCK TRACER TIP

One way to conduct a mock tracer on a product recall is to look at the last item that was recalled in the organization and trace how the response to the recall unfolded. Things to look at include how the recall notice entered the organization, who managed the recall, and how the product was removed from circulation.

to medical equipment recalls. The physician cannot articulate how the process works or identify a specific individual within the organization who is in charge of the product recall process. This prompts the surveyor to examine the issue further.

(Bracketed numbers correlate to Sample Tracer Questions on page 85.)

➡ *On a Patient Care Unit.* After speaking with the physician, the surveyor stops a nurse who is carrying an armful of supplies. "Do you know if this organization has a process in place for responding to a product recall?" asks the surveyor. The nurse looks a bit confused, and so the surveyor further expands the question. "What I mean is, let's say those supplies you're holding are recalled. Do you know how you would learn about that recall and who you would work with to remove the supplies from patient use?" [1–7] "Hmmm, I've never really thought about that," says the nurse. "I know the safety officer does some stuff with recalls—mostly supplies I think, and I think the biomedical equipment department does, too—for medical equipment—but I don't know the specifics. Maybe you should ask them?"

The surveyor asks the nurse about any training or orientation she's received on the product recall process, but the nurse cannot recall having any such training. [8]

➡ *At the Safety Officer's Office.* After speaking with the nurse, the surveyor proceeds to the safety officer's office, where she asks for a copy of the organization's policies on product recalls. The safety officer admits that he is not aware of any formal policies for recalls. The surveyor then asks the safety officer to describe the organization's process for responding to a product recall. [9–18] She asks about the types of products that would fall within a recall program—such as medical equipment, pharmaceuticals, and supplies. She then asks who has responsibility for the process of product recalls and how the organization ensures that recalled products are removed from circulation.

The safety officer explains, "I work with product recalls when I receive them. These are usually for supplies and such. I know my colleagues in the biomedical equipment and warehousing departments respond to recalls when they receive them as well, but there isn't one person in charge of this process." Based on this response, the surveyor spends some time talking with the safety officer about the benefits of an organizationwide, integrated program.

➡ *In the Biomedical Equipment Department.* The surveyor makes another stop at the biomedical equipment department, where she speaks with the manager. The manager outlines a detailed process that the biomedical equipment department uses for responding to medical equipment recall notices. The surveyor presses for more information on how this process works, who's in charge of it, and what products are included. Although the process seems sound, it deals only with medical equipment and does not involve any other areas in the organization. There does not seem to be any interdepartmental collaboration on this topic. [9–18]

➡ *At the Office of a Senior Leader.* The surveyor stops by the office of one of the organization's senior leaders. She mentions that she is concerned that the organization has no formal, collaborative, interdepartmental process for responding to product recalls, and she feels this could put the organization at risk.

➡ *Moving Forward.* Based on the tracer, the surveyor might follow up with a discussion on having the senior leadership work with the safety officer, biomedical equipment manager, and warehouse manager to develop a comprehensive recall response process and train staff on that process. In this way, the organization can work together to prevent overlooked recalls that could result in patient harm.

At-a-glance
- - - - - - - - - -
Compliance Strategies

Recalls and alerts can enter an organization in a number of ways, such as via physicians, through administrators, and through vendors. No matter how they enter, an organization must have a clear, centralized process for dealing with recalls and alerts, and all staff members should be familiar with this process. The process should specify how appropriate departments are notified of a recall or an alert and how the individuals responsible for safety within the organization review the recall of any products used within the organization.

Scenario 5-2.
Sample Tracer Questions

The bracketed numbers before each question correlate to questions, observations, and data review described in the sample tracer for Scenario 5-2. You can use the tracer worksheet form in Appendix B to develop a mock tracer (*see* an example of a completed tracer worksheet at the end of this section). The information gained by conducting a mock tracer can help to highlight a good practice and/or determine issues that may require further follow-up.

Physician/Nurse on the Patient Care Unit

[1]   Does the organization have a process for responding to product recalls?

[2]   Who is in charge of the product recall process?

[3]   What types of items could be recalled?

[4]   How do you become aware of a product recall?

[5]   What responsibilities do you have for product recalls?

[6]   What process do you follow when a piece of equipment, a medication, or a supply is recalled?

[7]   Who would you work with to remove the supplies from use?

[8]   What training and orientation have you received on the product recall process?

Safety Officer and Biomedical Equipment Manager

[9]   Describe the organization's policies for responding to a product recall.

[10] What types of products fall within a recall program?

[11] Has anyone been designated to provide oversight for the recall program?

[12] Who receives recall notices?

[13] What is done with these recall notices?

[14] How do you follow up on potential issues?

[15] Does any leadership-level group monitor recall activities?

[16] What inventories do you check when you receive a recall notice?

[17] Are inventories in care units ever checked or followed up on?

[18] How do you ensure that recalled products are removed from circulation?

SCENARIO 5-3. Responding to a Safe Medical Devices Act (SMDA) Incident

Summary

In the following scenario, a surveyor traces how an organization responds to a medical equipment failure that seriously harms a patient. Within the tracer, the surveyor explores issues relating to these priority focus areas:

- Equipment Use
- Orientation and Training
- Patient Safety

Scenario

In reviewing the minutes of an organization's EC committee meetings, a surveyor notes that a medical equipment failure that harmed a patient occurred within the past three months. The surveyor decides to trace the organization's response to this event.

(Bracketed numbers correlate to Sample Tracer Questions on pages 86–87.)

➡ *On the Patient Care Unit.* The surveyor first visits the unit on which the incident occurred and asks to speak to a physician involved in the incident. He asks the physician to describe the entire event, including what caused it, the impact on the patient, the medical equipment involved, how the clinical staff responded, how they notified the biomedical equipment department, and how they isolated the equipment. [1–6]

"How did you address the safety of the patient?" asks the surveyor. [7] "We have emergency clinical interventions that we follow during an emergency such as this," says the physician. "In this case, a nurse on the care team hand-ventilated the patient until we could get a new piece of equipment in place. Unfortunately, we did not have another piece of equipment readily available, and so we were hand-ventilating for awhile, and this caused the patient some distress."

The surveyor asks the physician about any training or orientation he has received on emergency clinical interventions, such as the one used during this incident. [8] The physician describes some regularly occurring education opportunities on this topic.

The surveyor and physician further discuss the incident and brainstorm some ways the organization could prevent such an occurrence in the future.

➡ *In the Biomedical Equipment Department.* After speaking with the physician, the surveyor goes to the biomedical equipment department, where he speaks to the manager there about the incident. He probes for information on how the clinical staff notified the biomedical equipment department, what the immediate response of the biomedical equipment department was to the incident, what the long-term response was, whether an investigation was conducted, and how the incident was reported to the appropriate authorities. [9–17]

MOCK TRACER TIP

Although an organization may never have had an event involving medical equipment failure, it is still helpful to perform a mock tracer to address this issue. This type of event could also be incorporated into an escalating emergency management (EM) drill, to see how an organization would respond to a medical equipment failure resulting, for example, from a power outage.

At-a-glance
Compliance Strategies

If a piece of equipment is thought to have caused or contributed to an event that results in patient harm, the SMDA requires that the problem be classified as a device failure or a device-related event. These terms are defined as follows:

- *Device failure:* Failure of a device to perform or function as intended, including any deviations from the device's performance specifications or intended use

- *Device-related event:* An event that could involve a device operating incorrectly, failing due to loss of some facilitywide system (such as electricity) or being temporarily affected by environmental factors (such as electromagnetic interference)

Organizations should keep these definitions in mind when completing any SMDA–related investigations involving faulty medical equipment.

How did you report the incident?" asks the surveyor. "Since there was some patient harm involved with the incident, we decided to go ahead and report it," says the biomedical equipment manager. "Ultimately, the patient was fine, but we felt that reporting what happened would be beneficial for us as well as other organizations. Completing the report was definitely a joint effort between biomedical equipment and risk management. We worked together to conduct an internal investigation, write up a report, and submit it to the U.S. Food and Drug Administration (FDA) through the SMDA Web site." The surveyor presses for details about this process, asking for information on how the two departments worked together, how they involved the legal department, and how they communicated with the clinical staff. He also asks to review the final report on the incident. [18–20]

The surveyor then asks the biomedical equipment manager how he thinks this incident could be prevented in the future. [21] They discuss various strategies for proactively reducing the risks associated with this equipment and its potential failure.

➡ *In the Risk Management Department.* Finally, the surveyor visits the risk management department, where he discusses the incident with a manager there. He asks for her perspective on the incident, focusing on her opinions about how well the various departments responded to the incident. He probes for information about the report that was submitted to the FDA and how that report was generated. [22–25]

➡ *Moving Forward.* Based on the tracer, the surveyor might follow up with a discussion with the risk manager about creating a root cause analysis team to further investigate the incident and identify ways to prevent such incidents in the future. [26]

Scenario 5-3.
Sample Tracer Questions

The bracketed numbers before each question correlate to questions, observations, and data review described in the sample tracer for Scenario 5-3. You can use the tracer worksheet form in Appendix B to develop a mock tracer (*see* an example of a completed tracer worksheet at the end of this section). The information gained by conducting a mock tracer can help to highlight a good practice and/or determine issues that may require further follow-up.

Physician on the Unit

[1]   Describe the event in which a piece of medical equipment failed.

[2]   What was the impact of this failure on the patient?

[3]   What circumstances led to the event?

[4]   How did the clinical staff respond to the event?

[5]   How did you notify the biomedical equipment department about the event?

[6]   How did you isolate the equipment?

[7]   How did you address the safety of the patient?

[8]   What training or orientation have you had on emergency clinical interventions such as the one used during this incident?

Biomedical Equipment Manager

[9]   How did the clinical staff notify the biomedical equipment department about the incident?

[10] What was the immediate response to the incident?

[11] What was the long-term response?

[12] Did the organization conduct an investigation?

[13] How was that investigation conducted?

[14] Who was involved in the investigation?

[15] Did the organization report the incident?

[16] To whom did the organization report it?

[17] How did the organization report it?

[18] How did biomedical equipment department and risk management department work together to create the report?

[19] How did the organization involve the legal department?

[20] How did you communicate with clinical staff?

[21] How could an event like this be prevented in the future?

Risk Manager

[22] How did the organization respond to the incident?

[23] Were you satisfied with the response?

[24] How well did the various departments work together?

[25] How did the organization generate the report for the FDA?

[26] Did the organization conduct a root cause analysis on this incident?

SCENARIO 5-4. Sterilizer Maintenance

Summary

In the following scenario, a surveyor traces how an organization conducts maintenance for sterilizers. Within the tracer, the surveyor explores issues relating to these priority focus areas:

• Equipment Use
• Orientation and Training
• Patient Safety
• Infection Control

Scenario

During the EC session at a large tertiary care center, a surveyor asks to see the organization's sterilizer maintenance policy as well as the sterilizers' Instructions for Use (IFU)—the equipment manual developed by the manufacturer and the FDA. After reviewing these documents, the surveyor notes that the organization's sterilizer maintenance policy does not match the manufacturer's recommendations nor does the organization have a standardized process for sterilizer maintenance. This triggers the need for a second generation tracer. This scenario is an example of a second generation tracer, which takes an in-depth look at a high-risk topic (*see* "Introduction," page 2).

(Bracketed numbers correlate to Sample Tracer Questions on page 89.)

➡ *In the Sterile Processing Department.* The surveyor first meets with the manager of the sterile processing department, asking what the manager knows about sterilizer maintenance activities. During this conversation, the surveyor is trying to determine if the manager understands how the sterilizers should be maintained, who is in charge of that maintenance activity, and how communication with that department occurs. [1–5]

"How does a sterilizer in this department receive appropriate maintenance?" asks the surveyor.

"The biomedical equipment department is in charge of maintaining our sterilizers," says the manager. "When maintenance is scheduled, someone from the department comes here, performs the maintenance, performance-tests the machine, and releases it back to us for use. Before using the sterilizer, I perform another set of parametric, chemical, and biological tests to double check that the equipment is functioning properly."

The surveyor then asks for details about repair efforts: How does the sterile processing department determine if a sterilizer is malfunctioning and needs repair? How does the department communicate with the biomedical equipment department about that repair? Is the equipment failure documented? Does a representative from the biomedical equipment department come on site at regular intervals or just when the sterilizers malfunction? [6–9]

→ *Office of the Biomedical Equipment Manager.* The next stop is the office of the biomedical equipment manager, who is in charge of the organization's medical equipment man-

agement program. The surveyor probes for information about how the department performs maintenance on the sterilizers, asking for details about the steps involved in maintenance efforts, who conducts the maintenance, the training these individuals receive, and how often the training occurs. He also asks how frequently the department performs preventive maintenance and what they do if a sterilizer fails a performance test on a visit. [10–16]

Next, the surveyor asks about the IFU recommendations for maintaining the sterilizers, including the manufacturer's recommendations regarding preventive maintenance. The biomedical equipment manager is not familiar with these recommendations nor can he fully describe the organization's policy for sterilizer maintenance. The surveyor and biomedical equipment manager discuss the IFU requirements and why meeting those requirements is critical to ensuring the safety of patients. [17]

In addition to questions about maintenance, the surveyor asks about repair efforts, including how the biomedical equipment department receives repair requests from the different units housing sterilizers, including the sterile processing department; how the biomedical equipment department ensures timely repairs; and whether those repairs are documented. [18–20]

At the close of this conversation, the surveyor stresses the need to update the sterilizer maintenance policy and verify that practice matches the new policy. The surveyor and manager talk about how to develop a standardized process for sterilizer maintenance, with the surveyor suggesting that the organization form a task force to review and address the issue. He suggests that the task force consult not only the IFU recommendations but also the Association for the Advancement of Medical Instrumentation (AAMI) recommendations. The surveyor emphasizes the need for training associated with the new standardized process to make sure all sterilizers are maintained and repaired appropriately.

→ *Office of the Facility Manager.* The surveyor next goes to the office of the facility manager, where the surveyor asks about how the organization ensures the adequate supply of quality steam for the sterilizers. The facility manager and the surveyor discuss the importance of quality steam in an effective steam sterilization process. During this conversation, the surveyor probes for information about the dryness of the steam and the level of noncondensable gas in the steam. The facility manager indicates that steam dryness follows AAMI recommendations and is between 97% and 100% with non-

MOCK TRACER TIP

As with other types of tracers, organizations can perform mock second generation tracers. This is done by deeply exploring a high-risk topic in detail. When conducting mock tracers, look for challenging tracer subjects that might present opportunities to go in-depth, such as cleaning, disinfection, and sterilization; contracted services; and other topics. Explore all aspects of a topic and follow that topic to different departments, asking questions that will ultimately foster a thorough and comprehensive exploration.

At-a-glance
Compliance Strategies

In hospitals, sterilizers may be found in sterile processing, laboratory, and surgery areas. Individuals in charge of an organization's medical equipment management program should have open lines of communication with the staff members responsible for performance testing sterilizers in these areas to help anticipate any problems with sterilizers and ensure that any problems that do arise are quickly resolved.

Standards in the "Infection Prevention and Control" (IC) chapter address the topic of performance testing sterilizers. Individuals in charge of medical equipment maintenance should familiarize themselves with these standards to be fully knowledgeable about the equipment.

condensable gas maintained at a level that will not impair steam penetration into sterilization loads. [21–23]

The surveyor follows up this exchange with questions about steam pipe insulation and design, verifying that they meet AAMI recommendations as well. Next, the surveyor presses for information on how steam quality is maintained and whether the organization has processes for monitoring and controlling steam generation; maintaining steam traps, boilers, and generators; and periodically assessing sterilization loads to support proper sterilizer performance. [24–25]

➜ *Moving Forward.* Based on the tracer, the surveyor might follow up with a discussion with the facility manager about the lack of standardized maintenance policy and the need for the facility manager to be a part of the task force to update and implement the new policy and associated training efforts, since this issue is so important in preserving the safety of patients.

Scenario 5-4.
Sample Tracer Questions

The bracketed numbers before each question correlate to questions, observations, and data review described in the sample tracer for Scenario 5-4. You can use the tracer worksheet form in Appendix B to develop a mock tracer (*see* an example of a completed tracer worksheet at the end of this section). The information gained by conducting a mock tracer can help to highlight a good practice and/or determine issues that may require further follow-up.

Manager of the Sterile Processing Department

[1] How does a sterilizer in this department receive appropriate maintenance?

[2] Who is in charge of sterilizer maintenance efforts?

[3] How do you communicate with the department in charge of maintenance efforts?

[4] How often should the sterilizers be maintained?

[5] Does the sterile processing department have access to the sterilizer maintenance records?

[6] How do you determine if a sterilizer is malfunctioning and needs repair?

[7] How do you communicate with the biomedical equipment department about the repair?

[8] Is the equipment failure documented? If so, how?

[9] Does a representative from the biomedical equipment department come on site at regular intervals or just when the sterilizers malfunction?

Manager of the Biomedical Equipment Department

[10] Is sterilizer maintenance part of the organization's overall medical equipment management program?

[11] What are the steps involved in sterilizer maintenance?

[12] Who conducts the maintenance?

[13] What training do these individuals receive?

[14] How often does training occur?

[15] How frequently is preventive maintenance performed?

[16] How do you respond when a sterilizer fails a performance test on a unit?

[17] What are the IFU recommendations for maintaining sterilizers? Why is it important to be familiar with these recommendations?

[18] How do you receive repair requests from the different units, including sterile processing?

[19] How do you ensure timely repairs?

[20] Are repairs documented? If so, how?

Facility Manager

[21] Why is steam quality important for sterilizers?

[22] How does the organization ensure the adequate supply of quality steam?

[23] What is the appropriate level of dryness? Gas concentration?

[24] Discuss the steam pipe insulation. How does the organization's piping meet AAMI recommendations?

[25] What processes are in place for maintaining steam quality; monitoring and controlling steam generation; maintaining steam traps, boilers, and generators; and periodically assessing sterilization loads to support proper sterilizer performance?

Sample Tracer Worksheet: Scenario 5-4.

The worksheet below is an example of how organizations can use the sample tracer questions for Scenario 5-4 in a worksheet format during a mock tracer. Scenario 5-4 is an example of a second generation tracer, which takes an in-depth look at a high-risk topic (see "Introduction," page 2). The bracketed numbers before each question correlate to questions described in the scenario. A **correct answer** is an appropriate answer that meets the requirements of the organization and other governing bodies. An **incorrect answer** should always include recommendations for follow-up.

Tracer Team Member(s): Art Cavanaugh
Subjects Interviewed: Saneetha Walker, Ted Drew, Michael Walks
Tracer Topic: Sterilizer maintenance

Data Record(s): logs of sterilizer maintenance
Unit(s) or Department(s): Central supply, biomedical equipment department, office of the facility manager

Interview Subject: Manager of the Sterile Processing Department

Questions	Correct Answer	Incorrect Answer	Follow-Up Needed	Comments or Notes
[1] How does a sterilizer in this department receive appropriate maintenance?	✓			Can describe basic process for sterilizer maintenance.
[2–3] Who is in charge of sterilizer maintenance efforts? How do you communicate with the department in charge of maintenance efforts?		✓	Form a multidisciplinary group to work on improving communication between departments that use sterilizers and the biomedical equipment department.	Identifies the biomedical equipment department but indicates that communication with this department could be better.
[4–5] How often should the sterilizers be maintained? Does the sterile processing department have access to the sterilizer maintenance records?		✓	Consider providing education to departments using sterilizers about maintenance frequency and documentation.	Not aware of the specifics regarding sterilizer maintenance, such as how often it should occur and how it is documented.
[6–7, 9] How do you determine if a sterilizer is malfunctioning and needs repair? How do you communicate with the biomedical equipment department about the repair? Does a representative from the biomedical equipment department come on site at regular intervals or just when the sterilizers malfunction?	✓		Follow up with biomedical equipment on their processes for repair and encourage them to enhance communication with departments using sterilizers.	Could describe what to do in the case of sterilizer malfunction and whom to call.

Interview Subject: Manager of the Sterile Processing Department (continued)				
Questions	**Correct Answer**	**Incorrect Answer**	**Follow-Up Needed**	**Comments or Notes**
[8] Is the equipment failure documented? If so, how?	✓			Shows me the log book where equipment failures are documented.

Interview Subject: Manager of the Biomedical Equipment Department				
Questions	**Correct Answer**	**Incorrect Answer**	**Follow-Up Needed**	**Comments or Notes**
[10–11] Is sterilizer maintenance part of the organization's overall medical equipment management program? What are the steps involved in sterilizer maintenance?		✓	Suggest forming a multidisciplinary team to work on standardizing the sterilizer maintenance effort. This team should review IFU and AAMI recommendations.	Although sterilizers are listed on the medical equipment inventory, sterilizer maintenance does not appear to be standardized.
[12–14] Who conducts the maintenance? What training do these individuals receive? How often does training occur?		✓	Provide further training for those individuals charged with sterilizer maintenance.	There are specific individuals who maintain the sterilizers, and they received initial training. However, there has been little continuing education or review of skills.
[15] How frequently is preventive maintenance performed?		✓	Again, recommend multidisciplinary group address this issue.	Could not describe a standardized process with regular preventive maintenance intervals.
[16] What are the IFU recommendations for maintaining sterilizers? Why is it important to be familiar with these recommendations?		✓	Underscore the importance of these recommendations in ensuring patient safety.	Could not describe the IFU's recommendations.
[17–20] How do you respond when a sterilizer fails a performance test on a unit? How do you receive repair requests from the different units, including sterile processing? How do you ensure timely repairs? Are repairs documented? If so, how?	✓		Recommend enhancing communication with departments that use sterilizers.	Seems to have the emergency repair process well in hand.

(continued)

Interview Subject: Facility Manager				
Questions	**Correct Answer**	**Incorrect Answer**	**Follow-Up Needed**	**Comments or Notes**
[21] Why is steam quality important for sterilizers?	✓			Very knowledgeable about the importance of steam in a safe sterilization process.
[22–23] How does the organization ensure the adequate supply of quality steam? What is the appropriate level of dryness? Gas concentration?	✓			Could describe processes for ensuring adequate supply and good quality, as well as appropriate dryness and gas concentration.
[24] Discuss the steam pipe insulation. How does the organization's piping meet AAMI recommendations?	✓			Could describe how pipes are insulated and whether they meet AAMI recommendations.
[25] What processes are in place for maintaining steam quality; monitoring and controlling steam generation; maintaining steam traps, boilers, and generators; and periodically assessing sterilization loads to support proper sterilizer performance?		✓	Closely review the processes for maintaining steam traps, boilers, and generators as well as processes for periodically assessing sterilization loads. These could be updated and refreshed.	Although he could describe many of these processes, there were some—such as periodically assessing sterilization loads—that could use review.

Tracer Scenarios for
UTILITIES

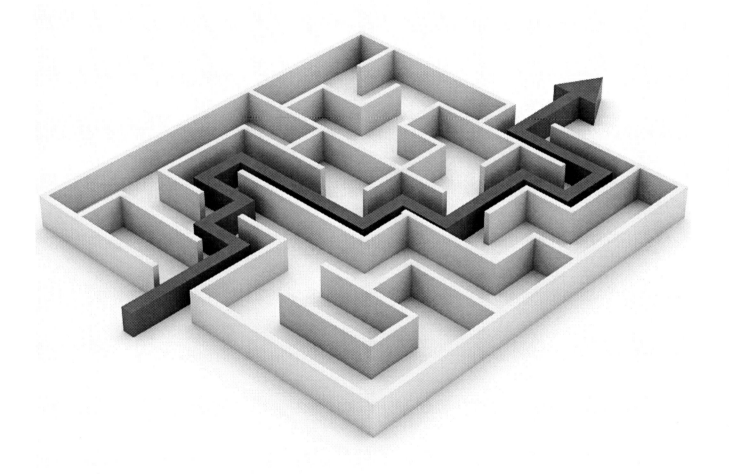

NOTE: No Two Tracers Are the Same

Please keep in mind that each tracer is unique. There is no way to know all of the questions that might be asked or documents that might be reviewed during a tracer—or what all the responses to the questions and documents might be. The possibilities are limitless, depending on the tracer topic and the organization's circumstances. These tracer scenarios and sample questions are provided as educational or training tools for organization staff; they are not scripts for real or mock tracers.

Section Elements

This section includes sample tracers—called scenarios—relevant to utilities. The section is organized as follows:

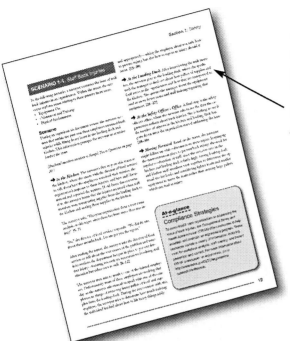

Scenarios: Each scenario presents what might happen when a surveyor conducts a specific type of tracer. The scenarios are presented in an engaging narrative format in which the reader "follows" the surveyor through the tracer scenario. Within the narrative are bracketed numbers that correspond to numbered sample tracer questions following the tracer.

Sample Tracer Questions: After each scenario narrative is a list of sample questions a surveyor might ask during that scenario. These questions can be used to develop and conduct mock tracers in your organization on topics similar to those covered in the scenario.

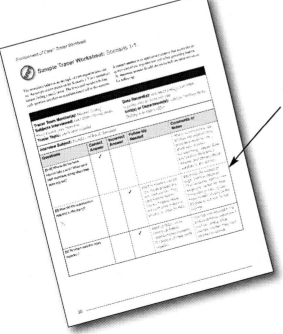

Sample Tracer Worksheet: At the end of the section is a sample worksheet that shows how the sample tracer questions for one select scenario in the section might be used in a worksheet format. The example shows how the worksheet might be completed as part of a tracer for that scenario. A blank form of the worksheet is available in Appendix B.

SCENARIO 6-1. Utility Outages

Summary

In the following scenario, a surveyor traces the activities that occurred during an organization's most recent utility failure. Within the tracer, the surveyor explores issues relating to these priority focus areas:

- Communication
- Equipment Use
- Orientation and Training
- Patient Safety
- Physical Environment

Scenario

During a patient tracer, as a surveyor is chatting with a nurse, the staff member mentions that the facility recently lost power because the utility company inadvertently cut a power line to the organization. Curious about the response to this incident, the surveyor decides to trace the utility failure, looking at all the activities that occurred during the event.

(Bracketed numbers correlate to Sample Tracer Questions on pages 96–97.)

→ *On the Unit.* To begin the tracer, the surveyor chats further with the nurse about the incident, asking her when it occurred and what happened. He probes for details about how the nurse responded to the event and ensured the safety of the patients under her care. [1–4]

"Were any patients harmed as a result of this outage?" asks the surveyor. [5] "Not that I know of," says the nurse. "Definitely not in this unit. I don't know what happened in the operating room down the hall, though. In here, all of our critical systems—life support, emergency lighting, and so on—transferred smoothly to emergency power, so we were able to keep things going relatively easily. The only thing was that the power was out for seven hours, so we had to live with the outage for awhile." [6–7]

The surveyor probes for more details on what was done to preserve patient safety during the seven hours of the outage. He also asks how communication between the unit and the power plant occurred and whether that communication was adequate. Finally, he asks about training and education regarding power outages and whether the nurse felt that the training and education adequately prepared her for the incident. [8–11]

→ *In the Operating Room.* Next, the surveyor visits the operating room (OR) and talks with the manager on duty there about the power outage. He asks if patients were affected by the outage, including whether anyone was in surgery at the time of the incident. [12–13] The manager explains that one patient was in the middle of surgery.

"How did OR staff ensure the safety of this patient?" asks the surveyor. [14] "The emergency power kicked in right away, and the patient was never in danger," says the manager. "The operating team brought the procedure to a stopping point and closed the patient quickly and safely. The patient was then taken to the intensive care unit for monitoring until the main power went back on and the surgery could resume. We notified the family immediately about what was going on and what we were doing to ensure that their loved one remained safe."

At-a-glance
Compliance Strategies

Automatic transfer switches are a critical component of a health care organization's emergency electrical distribution system. These electromechanical switchgears transfer the power from the utility to the emergency generator(s) in the event of an electrical outage. Upon the loss of power, the transfer switch signals the generator to start. When the generator gets up to speed and produces the proper voltage and frequency, the transfer switch transfers the load to the generator.

To ensure the smooth transfer to emergency power, organizations should test automatic transfer switches 12 times a year, at intervals not less than 20 days and not more than 40 days apart, following manufacturer instructions. Transfer switch testing is usually coordinated with a generator run test. In systems with multiple transfer switches, a different switch should be used to initiate the generator start each time until all switches have been tested.

Caution should be used when testing transfer switches, as they are potentially dangerous. Staff should receive training and wear appropriate personal protective equipment (PPE) during this activity.

The surveyor follows up on some further details about the event and also asks how the OR rearranged its surgery schedule to account for the lack of power. He then inquires about training and education regarding power failures. [15–17]

➡️ *At the Organization's Power Plant.* Finally, the surveyor stops by the organization's power plant and talks to the utilities manager who is in charge of the electrical system for the organization. They converse about the power outage and the events leading up to the outage. [18] In this conversation, the surveyor tries to determine whether emergency power worked as expected and whether there were areas that were supposed to be under emergency power that weren't. He also probes for information on the effectiveness of the organization's transfer switches and whether they are regularly tested. [19–22]

The utilities manager describes the incident in detail, including how well the emergency power functioned. He mentions that an area in one of the units that was supposed to be under emergency power didn't transfer over, and he had to bring up a small generator to power critical systems in the unit. Fortunately, there were no patients harmed because of the failure to transfer, and the organization has since addressed this issue so that during the next power failure, those systems will go on emergency power automatically. The surveyor asks if there were any other glitches in the power system and what is being done to address those glitches. [23–24]

Next, the surveyor asks for information about how the power plant communicated with organization staff regarding the status of the power outage and when power might be restored. They have a quick conversation about the organization's emergency management incident command center and whether it was activated during the outage. [25–27]

MOCK TRACER TIP

When performing a mock tracer on issues associated with the emergency power system, an organization may want to spend some time reviewing documentation. When done well, this documentation can show that the organization is diligent about testing its components of emergency power. When done poorly, this documentation can signal a deeper problem.

➡️ *Moving Forward.* Finally, the surveyor asks how the organization's power plant staff communicated with the power company and whether they had an established relationship before the incident. He asks the manager his opinion about why the outage occurred and whether a better relationship with the power company could have prevented the incident. [28–31] The surveyor encourages the utilities manager to have regular meetings with the power company to discuss possible ways to limit power outages and respond effectively to outages that do occur.

Scenario 6-1.
Sample Tracer Questions

The bracketed numbers before each question correlate to questions, observations, and data review described in the sample tracer for Scenario 6-1. You can use the tracer worksheet form in Appendix B to develop a mock tracer (*see* an example of a completed tracer worksheet at the end of this section). The information gained by conducting a mock tracer can help to highlight a good practice and/or determine issues that may require further follow-up.

Nurse on a Patient Care Unit

[1]   When did the power outage occur?

[2]   Describe the incident.

[3]   How did the organization respond to the power outage?

[4]   How did you ensure the safety of the patients under your care?

[5]   Were any patients harmed as a result of this outage?

[6]   What systems transferred to emergency power?

[7]   How smooth was that transfer?

[8]   What was done to preserve patient safety during the outage?

[9]   Describe the communication between the organization's power plant and this unit?

[10] What training and education regarding power outages have you received?

[11] Do you feel that this training and education adequately prepared you for the incident?

OR Manager

[12] Were patients affected by the power outage?

[13] Was anyone in surgery at the time?

[14] How did OR staff ensure the safety of anyone in surgery at the time of the outage?

[15] How did the department rearrange the schedule for the OR?

[16] What training and education have OR staff received on power outages?

[17] Is that training effective?

Utilities Manager

[18] Describe the power outage and the events leading up to it.

[19] Did emergency power work as expected?

[20] How well did the transfer switches work?

[21] Had the organization recently tested the transfer switches?

[22] Were there areas that were supposed to be under emergency power that weren't?

[23] What other glitches occurred during the outage?

[24] How has the organization addressed those glitches?

[25] How did this department communicate with patient care units about the outage and when power would be restored?

[26] Did the organization activate its incident command center? If not, why not?

[27] How did the process work?

[28] How did the organization communicate with the power company?

[29] Does the organization have an established relationship with the power company?

[30] What does the organization do to sustain that relationship?

[31] What is the organization doing to prevent this type of situation in the future?

SCENARIO 6-2. Generator Testing

In the following scenario, a surveyor traces an organization's generator testing activities. Within the tracer, the surveyor explores issues relating to these priority focus areas:

- Communication
- Equipment Use
- Orientation and Training
- Patient Safety
- Physical Environment

Scenario

When reviewing documentation during the Environment of Care (EC) session, a surveyor notes that an organization has not performed the necessary emergency generator tests within the time frames established in the EC standards. Curious about this issue, the surveyor decides to do a tracer on the topic.

(Bracketed numbers correlate to Sample Tracer Questions on pages 98–99.)

➡ *At the EC Office.* The surveyor starts the tracer in the EC office, asking the manager in charge of the physical plant several questions about the organization's generator testing efforts.

"How often do you test your emergency backup generators?" asks the surveyor. [1] "Based on our organization's policy, we do it 6 times a year," says the manager. The surveyor discusses the fact that the Joint Commission EC standards require organizations to test 12 times a year, at intervals not less than 20 days and not more than 40 days apart.

The surveyor then asks how the organization initiates generator tests, what the process involved in ensuring that all tests are accomplished in a timely manner is, and why the organization's testing efforts do not currently comply with the standards. [2–4]

At-a-glance
- - - - - - - - - -
Compliance Strategies

In addition to testing emergency generators, an organization should also test battery-powered egress lights monthly for a minimum of 30 seconds and annually for a minimum of 90 minutes. An organization may choose to replace batteries annually instead of conducting the 90-minute test. If this option is selected, the organization should test 10% of the replacement batteries for the 90-minute duration. Required locations for this test include generator locations and new or renovated anesthetizing locations, such as ORs.

The manager explains, "We run the generators for at least 30 continuous minutes, and once every three years for at least four continuous hours. This not only allows us to ensure that the emergency power generator starts and runs properly but also that the unit's surrounding environment is appropriate and safe and that backup power will be available for the duration of an emergency. Although the 30-minute tests are important, the 4-hour tests provide a way to determine that our entire system is reliable." The surveyor asks for more details about these different tests, including the load under which each generator is tested. The surveyor queries the manager about what training and education the individuals in charge of generator testing receive. [5–7]

The surveyor then asks what the organization does to test the generator's fuel oil, track oil expiration dates, and replace stale fuel oil. He also asks about transfer switches—how often they are tested, how the organization coordinates transfer switch testing with generator testing, and how the organization ensures that every transfer switch is tested. [8–11]

➡ *Asking About Staff Preparedness.* The surveyor asks the manager in charge of the physical plant what the organization does to prepare staff throughout the facility for a generator test. He asks about any contingency plans associated with generator testing, including how patient care staff and administrative staff are informed of a pending test and are put on "standby" to implement power failure contingency plans. He then asks if the organization restricts its services during a generator test to minimize any patient impact. [12–14]

"Do you have a secondary generator unit that can be in place before each four-hour generator test?" [15] "Wow, that would be great, wouldn't it?" says the manager. "Unfortunately, our senior leadership would never give us the funds for that. They make it pretty clear that these tests are inconvenient for us all, and they want them to occur with as little fuss as possible." The surveyor discusses the fact that having a secondary generator would allow for a redundant system that will engage if the generator fails the test and a power outage occurs. He makes a note to speak to senior leadership about this topic.

➡ *On a Patient Care Unit.* The surveyor visits a patient care unit. He asks the nurse manager on duty if she had advance notice of the most recent emergency generator test and what happened during that test. He also asks whether she knows what to do if a test fails and power goes out. He queries the nurse manager about the risks involved in not testing generators regularly. [16–19] Although the nurse manager has some familiarity with the generator testing efforts, it is clear this is not an important issue for her or the organization.

➡ *At a Senior Leader's Office.* Finally, the surveyor stops by the office of a senior leader and asks about his familiarity with generator testing. The surveyor wants to determine whether the leader is aware of the importance of generator testing and why communication between departments during a test is critical. He also wants to determine whether the leader understands the need for a secondary backup generator to ensure patient safety if the power fails during the test of the main generator. [20–26]

➡ *Moving Forward.* At the conclusion of his conversation with the senior leader, the surveyor reiterates how to improve generator testing, including complying with the standards that require a specific frequency of tests and also suggests establishing better contingency plans.

MOCK TRACER TIP

When conducting a mock tracer on an organization's processes for generator testing, examine any contingency plans the organization has in place if the generator fails and the power goes out. In the middle of a utility failure is not the time to discover that a contingency plan is not effective or—even worse—nonexistent. Organizations that closely examine their contingency plans and address any problems with those plans are better prepared for an emergency and increase the likelihood of preserving patient safety and the quality of care.

Scenario 6-2.
Sample Tracer Questions

The bracketed numbers before each question correlate to questions, observations, and data review described in the sample tracer for Scenario 6-2. You can use the tracer worksheet form in Appendix B to develop a mock tracer (*see* an example of a completed tracer worksheet at the end of this section). The information gained by conducting a mock tracer can help to highlight a good practice and/or determine issues that may require further follow-up.

Manager of the Physical Plant

[1] How often does the organization test its emergency backup generators?

[2] How does the organization initiate generator tests?

[3] What is the process involved in ensuring that all tests are accomplished in a timely manner?

[4] How does the organization test its generators?

[5] Why is it important to do a 30-minute test and a four-hour test?

[6] Under what load does the organization test each generator?

[7] What training and education have the individuals in charge of generator testing received?

[8] What does the organization do to test the generator's fuel oil? track expiration dates? replace stale fuel oil?

[9] How often does the organization test transfer switches?

[10] How does the organization coordinate transfer switch testing with generator testing?

[11] How does the organization ensure that every transfer switch is tested?

[12] What does the organization do to prepare for a generator test?

[13] What contingency plans does the organization have in place in case the generator fails the test and the power goes out?

[14] Does the organization restrict its services during a generator test to minimize any patient impact?

[15] Does the organization have a secondary generator unit that can be in place before each four-hour generator test?

Nurse Manager

[16] When was the last time the organization did an emergency generator test?

[17] Were you notified ahead of time that the test would be happening?

[18] What contingency plans did your unit have in place in case the generator failed and the power went out?

[19] Why is it important to test the generators periodically?

Senior Leader

[20] Why does the organization do generator testing?

[21] How often does the organization do generator testing?

[22] Why is it important to test generators frequently?

[23] How well does the organization communicate about generator tests?

[24] Why is interdepartmental communication important before, during, and after these tests?

[25] Does the organization have a secondary backup generator in place in case the primary generator fails the test and the power goes out?

[26] Why is it important to have a secondary backup generator in place?

SCENARIO 6-3. Mapping Utilities

Summary

In the following scenario, a surveyor traces an organization's utilities map. Within the tracer, the surveyor explores issues relating to these priority focus areas:
- Orientation and Training
- Physical Environment

Scenario

As a surveyor talks to an organization's facilities manager, the subject of the organization's utilities comes up. Interested to see if the organization properly maps these utilities, the surveyor starts a tracer on the topic.

(Bracketed numbers correlate to Sample Tracer Questions on page 101.)

→ *At the Facilities Manager's Office.* To begin the tracer, the surveyor asks to see the organization's utilities map.

"What do these drawings show?" asks the surveyor. [1] "These drawings show the operations of all our different utilities systems, including the water, medical gas, electrical, and heating, cooling, and ventilating systems," says the facilities manager. "Specifically, these drawings show where all our utilities enter the building and how they are distributed throughout the facility. They also show where the endpoints of use are and where we can perform emergency interventions, if necessary."

The surveyor follows up this answer by asking how the drawings are created, who creates them, and how they are amended when necessary. He asks the facilities manager to verbally "walk through" one of the utility systems shown on the map. [2–5] In this conversation, the surveyor wants to ascertain whether the facilities manager understands the drawings and can use them as a reference during partial or complete emergency shutdowns.

The surveyor then asks how the facilities manager would shut down certain systems if an emergency intervention were necessary, including how he would notify staff in affected areas and how he would obtain emergency repair services. [6–8] The surveyor also asks about any training the facilities manager has had on utilities shutdowns and whether anyone else in the organization is qualified to shut down a utility during an emergency situation. The surveyor then probes for information about how the organization ensures that only qualified individuals can shut down utilities. [9–11]

➡️ *In the Building.* After thoroughly discussing the drawings and emergency shutdown procedures, the surveyor asks the facilities manager to give him a tour of the utilities systems and show him a sampling of how the organization labels utilities system controls to facilitate partial or complete emergency shutdowns. During this tour, the surveyor presses for information on how the controls are labeled, who labels them, and the process for changing labels when that is necessary. [12–14] He checks a few control labels against the utilities drawings to make sure they are labeled the same way in both places.

➡️ *On a Patient Care Unit.* The surveyor stops by a patient care unit and asks a physician on the unit what he would do in the event of a utility failure. To determine whether the physician understands and can fulfill his role during a utility failure, the surveyor presents a scenario involving a medical gas failure resulting in a loss of pressure to a ventilator. He follows up by asking what the physician would do to ensure the safety of patients. [19–21] In this conversation, the surveyor is trying to determine whether the physician understands his role during a utility failure and can fulfill that role, if necessary.

"Have you ever received training on how to respond to a medical gas failure?" asks the surveyor. [22] "I was at a medical conference a few months ago, and an organization did a presentation about how it had a medical gas failure and what the response to that failure was," says the physician. "I found it very beneficial, as I had never really thought of this type of emergency happening here. So, I spoke to our chief of medicine to see if we could have that organization come and talk at a medical staff meeting. I think they'll be here next month."

➡️ *Moving Forward.* After speaking with the physician and other staff on the patient care unit about utilities failures, the surveyor returns to the facilities manager's office, where he asks to see the organization's written procedures for responding to utilities system disruptions. He asks who creates these procedures and how often they are reviewed. He also asks about training and education on the procedures for both facilities staff and clinical staff. [15–18] In this conversation, he tries to determine whether training and education on this topic are adequate and how the organization can tell that it's sufficient and appropriate.

MOCK TRACER TIP

When performing a mock tracer about how an organization maps its utilities, it's important to have an understanding of staff education about utilities shutoffs. For example, do facilities staff members understand where to shut off a utility during a partial shutdown so as not to affect the entire utility system? It can be helpful to have staff demonstrate the right place to do a partial shutdown.

At-a-glance
Compliance Strategies

The label on a utility system control depends on the utility. For example, The Joint Commission expects organizations with piped medical gas systems to label their main and area supply shutoff valves, including a description of the gas type located in the system and the areas the system serves. It is good practice to check these labels for accuracy during an environmental tour. Organizations often change room designations and signage, and the room(s) or areas served by the shutoff valve might not be accurately reflected.

Scenario 6-3.
Sample Tracer Questions

The bracketed numbers before each question correlate to questions, observations, and data review described in the sample tracer for Scenario 6-3. You can use the tracer worksheet form in Appendix B to develop a mock tracer (*see* an example of a completed tracer worksheet at the end of this section). The information gained by conducting a mock tracer can help to highlight a good practice and/or determine issues that may require further follow-up.

Facilities Manager

[1] [Showing the facilities manager the utilities system drawings] Describe what these drawings show.

[2] Who created the drawings?

[3] How were they created?

[4] How are they amended when necessary?

[5] Verbally "walk through" one of the utilities systems shown on the map.

[6] How would you shut down a particular system on this map in the event of an emergency?

[7] How would you notify staff in affected areas?

[8] How would the organization obtain emergency repair services?

[9] What training have you received about utilities system shutdowns?

[10] Is anyone else in the organization qualified to shut down a utility during an emergency situation?

[11] How does the organization ensure that only qualified individuals can shut down utilities?

[12] Show a sample of how the organization labels utilities system controls to facilitate partial or complete emergency shutdowns.

[13] Who labels the controls?

[14] How are the labels changed if necessary?

[15] Show the organization's written procedures for responding to utilities system disruptions.

[16] Who creates these procedures?

[17] How often are they reviewed?

[18] Are facilities staff and clinical staff trained on these procedures?

Physician on a Patient Care Unit

[19] What would you do in the event of a utility failure, such as a medical gas failure?

[20] How would you ensure the safety of patients?

[21] How would you communicate with the facilities management department?

[22] Have you received training on how to respond to a utility failure?

SCENARIO 6-4. Heating, Ventilating, and Air-Conditioning (HVAC) Systems

Summary

In the following scenario, a surveyor traces an organization's heating, ventilating, and air-conditioning (HVAC) systems. Within the tracer, the surveyor explores issues relating to these priority focus areas:

- Communication
- Equipment Use
- Orientation and Training
- Physical Environment

Scenario

A surveyor is tracing the care of a patient in the neonatal intensive care unit (NICU). Because the dangers associated with infection in this area are significant, the surveyor begins looking at how the organization controls airborne contaminants in the unit. Specifically, she focuses on tracing the organization's HVAC system.

MOCK TRACER TIP

Airborne contaminants can include biological agents—bacteria, viruses, and molds—as well as gases, fumes, and construction-related dust. Preventing the spread of airborne contaminants is more than just an EC issue; it is also critical in preventing the spread of infection. Therefore, when tracing an HVAC system, EC professionals should consider involving infection preventionists in the tracer because they can serve as valuable resources on how the organization can best prevent the spread of infection.

(Bracketed numbers correlate to Sample Tracer Questions on page 103.)

➡ **In the NICU.** The surveyor asks a nurse in the NICU about the ventilation system in the area. **[1]** Although she does not expect the nurse to know all the details about the system, the surveyor wants to make sure the nurse has a basic understanding of how the system works and why it's important. The surveyor also wants to see if the staff member can recognize when the system is not operating appropriately and knows who to call about the problem. She asks about any training and education the nurse has received on the system. **[2–5]**

At-a-glance
Compliance Strategies

An organization's ventilation policies depend on the procedures it performs, the patients it serves, and the organisms it identifies. Different areas might require different levels of temperature, humidity, velocity, and filtration. For example, the Centers for Disease Control and Prevention (CDC) developed guidelines regarding appropriate ventilation for ORs. Following are some of the suggestions included in these guidelines:

- Maintain positive-pressure ventilation with respect to corridors and areas adjacent to the OR.

- Maintain at least 15 air changes per hour, with at least 3 of these being fresh air.

- Filter all recirculated and fresh air through appropriate filters to provide a minimum of 90% efficiency.

- In rooms not engineered for horizontal laminar air flow, introduce air at the ceiling and exhaust near the floor.

- Keep OR doors closed except for passage of equipment, personnel, and patients, and limit entry to essential personnel.

Pressure gradients and air-exchange rates should be designed and set according to the needs of the services performed as well as the individuals served.

➡ **In the Engineering Department.** The surveyor next visits a senior engineer in the organization and asks him several questions about the HVAC system.

"How old is the system?" asks the surveyor. **[6]** "It's five years old," says the engineer. "We installed it during a renovation of the main building. It was designed and installed based on the *Guidelines for Design and Construction of Hospitals and Health Care Facilities*. We contracted a credentialed design professional who adhered to specifications contained in our state and local codes as well as those from the American Society of Heating, Refrigerating and Air-Conditioning Engineers (ASHRAE)." **[7–8]**

"I assume that the system serves the entire facility. Are there any specific areas in which the system controls airborne contaminants?" asks the surveyor. **[9]** "Yes," says the engineer. "The system specifically addresses airborne contaminants in areas that treat individuals who are more highly susceptible to infection due to disease processes or immune status. For example, it services our ORs, special procedure rooms, delivery rooms, NICU, airborne infectious isolation rooms, protective isolation rooms, laboratories, and sterile supply rooms."

➡ **Asking About Readings.** The surveyor asks the engineer a series of questions about how the organization sets and maintains appropriate measures such as pressure relationships, air-exchange rates, filtration efficiencies, temperature, and humidity in the HVAC system. Basically, she wants to discover how the organization validates that the HVAC system is performing to design. **[10–14]**

Through her conversation with the senior engineer, the surveyor learns that much of the organization's monitoring efforts are automated. So the surveyor asks to see the control room, where she views several reports on the HVAC system. She asks the senior engineer to describe how he reads and responds to these reports. **[15–18]**

The surveyor then asks what happens if HVAC readings vary from the appropriate settings. The senior engineer describes an alarm system on the computer that sounds if a reading veers out of range. The surveyor presses for information about how the engineer would respond to an alarm and how the organization ensures that alarms are heard. **[19–22]**

➡ **Moving Forward.** Finally, the surveyor asks the senior engineer about the preventive maintenance, cleaning, and inspection schedules for the HVAC system, querying how the schedules are established and adhered to. The senior engineer says that most of the maintenance, testing, and cleaning are done by an outside contractor. The surveyor asks how the organization works with the contractor to ensure the best possible HVAC system. The surveyor also asks how the organization ensures the proper fit of filters and quick replacement of fans, coils, and belts, as these are critical items that cannot wait until routine maintenance to be fixed. [23–29]

Scenario 6-4.
Sample Tracer Questions

The bracketed numbers before each question correlate to questions, observations, and data review described in the sample tracer for Scenario 6-4. You can use the tracer worksheet form in Appendix B to develop a mock tracer (*see* an example of a completed tracer worksheet at the end of this section). The information gained by conducting a mock tracer can help to highlight a good practice and/or determine issues that may require further follow-up.

Nurse on a Patient Care Unit

[1] What can you tell me about the ventilation system in this area?

[2] Why is this ventilation system important?

[3] How can you tell if the system is working?

[4] What do you do if the system isn't working?

[5] What training and education have you received on this system?

Senior Engineer

[6] How old is the system?

[7] How did the organization ensure the proper design and installation of the system?

[8] What regulations govern the design and installation of the system?

[9] In what areas does the system control airborne contaminants?

[10] How does the organization set and maintain appropriate pressure relationships?

[11] How does the organization set and maintain appropriate air-exchange rates?

[12] How does the organization set and maintain appropriate filtration efficiencies?

[13] How does the organization set and maintain appropriate temperature and humidity?

[14] How does the organization validate that the HVAC system is performing to design?

[15] How does the automated system work?

[16] Who interprets the reports from the system?

[17] How do these people interpret the reports?

[18] How do they respond to those reports?

[19] What happens if pressure relationships, air-exchange rates, filtration efficiencies, temperature, and humidity vary from the appropriate settings?

[20] How does the alarm system work?

[21] How does the organization ensure that alarms are heard?

[22] How would you respond to an alarm?

[23] What kind of preventive maintenance does the organization do on the system?

[24] How does the organization keep the system clean?

[25] Who is in charge of that work?

[26] How does the organization adhere to an appropriate schedule for cleaning and maintenance?

[27] How does the organization work with the contractor to ensure the best possible HVAC system?

[28] How does the organization ensure the proper fit of filters?

[29] How does the organization ensure the quick replacement of fans, coils, and belts?

Sample Tracer Worksheet: Scenario 6-2.

The worksheet below is an example of how organizations can use the sample tracer questions for Scenario 6-2 in a worksheet format during a mock tracer. The bracketed numbers before each question correlate to questions described in the scenario.

A **correct answer** is an appropriate answer that meets the requirements of the organization and other governing bodies. An **incorrect answer** should always include recommendations for follow-up.

Tracer Team Member(s): Joseph Drend
Subjects Interviewed: Enrique Valdez, Jennifer Berry, Michael Janis
Tracer Topic: Generator testing

Data Record(s): generator set log; fuel quality log; test report; service records
Unit(s) or Department(s): EC unit, patient care unit 12A, senior leader's office

Interview Subject: Manager of the Physical Plant

Questions	Correct Answer	Incorrect Answer	Follow-Up Needed	Comments or Notes
[1] How often does the organization test its emergency backup generators?		✓	Need to conduct tests more frequently. Work with plant manager to increase the frequency of testing.	Organization only tests every other month. Standards require testing 12 times per year, at intervals not less than 20 days and not more than 40 days apart.
[2–3] How does the organization initiate generator tests? What is the process involved in ensuring that all tests are accomplished in a timely manner?		✓	Should create a schedule for testing and gain leadership support for regular testing. Maybe include this in the next EC committee meeting and brainstorm solutions.	Generator testing seems somewhat haphazard. The organization doesn't have a specific schedule in place.
[4–5] How does the organization test its generators? Why is it important to do a 30-minute test and a four-hour test?	✓			Describes appropriate testing methodology. Can describe benefits of both 30-minute tests and four-hour tests.
[6] Under what load does the organization test each generator?	✓			States that the organization tests using at least 30% load of nameplate to prevent "wet stacking." This is appropriate for diesel-powered generators.

Interview Subject: _Manager of the Physical Plant (continued)_				
Questions	**Correct Answer**	**Incorrect Answer**	**Follow-Up Needed**	**Comments or Notes**
[7] What training and education have the individuals in charge of generator testing received?		✓	Should review the training materials and make sure they talk about the frequency of generator testing and the importance of this frequency.	Describes both initial orientation and refresher training. Need to emphasize the need for more frequent tests in future training.
[8] What does the organization do to test the generator's fuel oil? track expiration dates? replace stale fuel oil?	✓			Able to describe procedures for testing fuel oil, tracking expiration dates, and replacing stale fuel oil.
[9–11] How often does the organization test transfer switches? How does the organization coordinate tests with generator testing? How does the organization ensure that every switch is tested?		✓	Should develop a system to make sure transfer switch testing occurs on schedule and tests all the different switches. Need to work to better coordinate this effort with generator testing.	The organization doesn't test transfer switches as often as required. Need to work on coordinating with generator testing.
[12] What does the organization do to prepare for a generator test?		✓	Should consider launching a performance improvement project to improve the frequency and coordination of generator testing. Should involve physical plant personnel as well as clinical staff and leadership in this effort.	Preparation efforts appear to be a little haphazard. Little to no coordination with patient care units, administrative staff, or leadership.
[13–15] What contingency plans does the organization have in place in case the generator fails the test and the power goes out? Does the organization restrict its services during generator tests to minimize patient impact? Does the organization have a secondary unit that can be put in place before each generator test?		✓	Need to create better contingency plans, including building awareness of patient care staff members about when the test will occur and what their responsibilities are if a test fails. Also, should seek funds for a supplemental generator.	Weak contingency plans. No supplemental generator in place. If generator failed the test and the power went out, could be problematic for the organization.

(continued)

105

Interview Subject: Nurse Manager

Questions	Correct Answer	Incorrect Answer	Follow-Up Needed	Comments or Notes
[16–18] When was the last time the organization did an emergency generator test? Were you notified ahead of time? What contingency plans did your unit have in place in case the generator failed and the power went out?		✓	Need to develop concrete contingency activities for staff to implement in case of emergency. Training and education on these contingencies is paramount.	Vaguely aware of generator test. Not sure what she would have done if power went out with no emergency power.
[19] Why is it important to test the generators periodically?		✓	Further education and training may be beneficial to at least build awareness of the roles and responsibilities of patient care staff during a generator test.	Cannot describe the reasons for frequent generator testing.

Interview Subject: Senior Leader

Questions	Correct Answer	Incorrect Answer	Follow-Up Needed	Comments or Notes
[20–22] Why does the organization do generator testing? How often does the organization do generator testing? Why is it important to test generators frequently?		✓	Need to build awareness among senior leadership of the importance of generator testing and how frequently it occurs. Should explain the consequences of not performing generator tests and of not having contingency plans in place.	Not all that familiar with the generator testing efforts of the organization. Cannot describe why this is so important. Assumes that all will work out fine. Feels that the likelihood of a generator failing a test and the power going out is slim and worth the risk.
[23–24] How well does the organization communicate about generator tests? Why is interdepartmental communication important before, during, and after these tests?		✓	Need to improve communication between physical plant staff and senior leadership around this topic and its importance.	Not aware of communication efforts before, during, and after the tests. Senior leader says, "I thought this was a maintenance issue. Why do I need to be involved?"

Interview Subject: *Senior Leader (continued)*				
Questions	**Correct Answer**	**Incorrect Answer**	**Follow-Up Needed**	**Comments or Notes**
[25–26] Does the organization have a secondary backup generator in place in case the primary generator fails the test and the power goes out? Why is it important to have a secondary backup generator in place?		✓	Need to educate leaders further on the importance and the need to designate funds for emergency backup.	Didn't understand the importance of a secondary backup generator until I explained the potential consequences of not having such a generator. I explained that the cost of renting a generator during the four-hour tests is far less than the costs involved in recovering from an emergency in which the power goes out and there is no backup power.

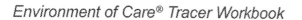

Tracer Scenarios for
MONITORING AND IMPROVING
PERFORMANCE

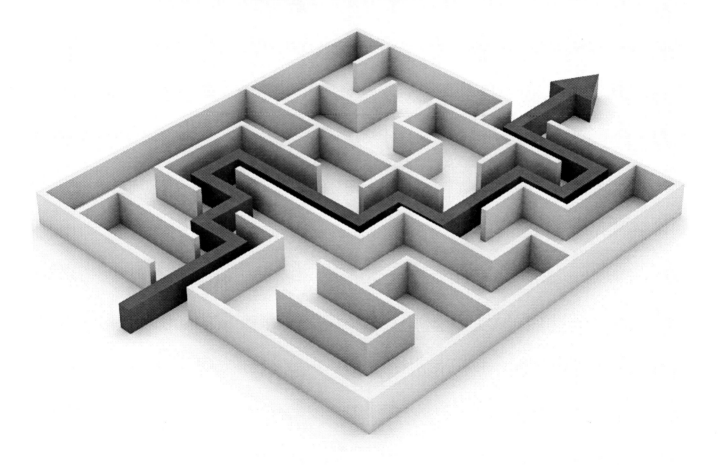

NOTE: No Two Tracers Are the Same

Please keep in mind that each tracer is unique. There is no way to know all of the questions that might be asked or documents that might be reviewed during a tracer—or what all the responses to the questions and documents might be. The possibilities are limitless, depending on the tracer topic and the organization's circumstances. These tracer scenarios and sample questions are provided as educational or training tools for organization staff; they are not scripts for real or mock tracers.

Section Elements

This section includes sample tracers—called scenarios—relevant to monitoring and improving performance. The section is organized as follows:

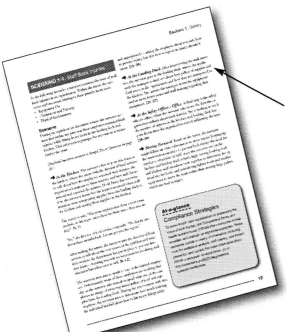

Scenarios: Each scenario presents what might happen when a surveyor conducts a specific type of tracer. The scenarios are presented in an engaging narrative format in which the reader "follows" the surveyor through the tracer scenario. Within the narrative are bracketed numbers that correspond to numbered sample tracer questions following the tracer.

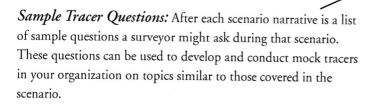

Sample Tracer Questions: After each scenario narrative is a list of sample questions a surveyor might ask during that scenario. These questions can be used to develop and conduct mock tracers in your organization on topics similar to those covered in the scenario.

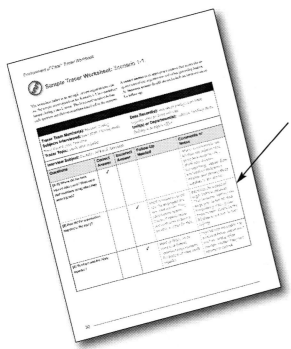

Sample Tracer Worksheet: At the end of the section is a sample worksheet that shows how the sample tracer questions for one select scenario in the section might be used in a worksheet format. The example shows how the worksheet might be completed as part of a tracer for that scenario. A blank form of the worksheet is available in Appendix B.

SCENARIO 7-1. Performance Monitors

Summary

In the following scenario, a surveyor traces how an organization selects and responds to performance monitors. Within the tracer, the surveyor explores issues relating to these priority focus areas:

- Communication
- Patient Safety
- Physical Environment
- Quality Improvement Activities

Scenario

While reviewing the minutes of an organization's environment of care (EC) committee meetings, a surveyor notes that the organization is trying to reduce the number of unauthorized after-hours entries into the building. The organization has experienced several security incidents involving unauthorized entries, including a few thefts. To help address this issue, the organization has designed a performance monitor that it uses to collect data and monitor performance over time. Curious about how the organization created this performance monitor and how it creates other such monitors, the surveyor decides to trace the topic.

(Bracketed numbers correlate to Sample Tracer Questions on page 112.)

➡️ *At the Office of the Safety Officer.* First, the surveyor stops in at the office of the safety officer to chat with him about the organization's approach to creating and maintaining performance monitors. [1–2] During this conversation, the surveyor asks about several different performance monitors, including the one related to the number of unauthorized after-hours entries. The surveyor asks how and why these performance monitors were created and how long they have been in use. [3–4] She follows up by asking what the different monitors measure and why collecting data on those topics is important. [5] In this conversation, she is trying to make sure the organization has really put some thought into its performance monitors.

Next, the surveyor asks about the methods of data collection associated with the monitors, specifically focusing on the number of unauthorized entries. [6] The safety officer explains, "Every time a security officer has to stop someone who shouldn't be there in the building after hours, he or she docu-

ments it on a form that the security department maintains. We combine those data with information from incident reports, including thefts, to come up with an overall number."

➡️ *Asking How Data Are Used.* The surveyor then questions the safety officer further for information on what the organization does with the data collected using the performance monitors. She asks how the organization responds to performance monitor data in general. [7]

She then asks how the safety officer uses performance monitor data to recommend EC–related improvement activities to organization leadership. Next, she asks how leadership prioritizes the performance improvement recommendations it receives from throughout the organization and makes selections from among them. [8–9]

"Do you document which performance improvement projects are selected for implementation during any given year?" asks the surveyor. [10] "Yes, because sometimes organization leaders don't select an EC process for review, but I still want to note that I made the recommendation and to describe why that process wasn't selected."

➡️ *In the Security Department.* The surveyor goes to the security department, where she asks the security manager how the department collects data for the performance monitor related to unauthorized after-hours access. He confirms that the department collects the data in the way the safety officer describes. [11]

MOCK TRACER TIP

When conducting a mock tracer on performance monitoring, it can be helpful to walk through an organization's most recent EC–related improvement initiative. Why did the organization choose to pursue this initiative? How did the organization approach it? How did the organization monitor performance? What did the organization do with the information collected? Also, look at the final results of the improvement project and whether the organization met its goals for improvement. Going through a step-by-step analysis via a mock tracer can help an organization determine whether it has an effective approach to performance monitoring and improvement.

"Do you have any documentation on that monitor?" asks the surveyor. [12–14] "Yes, we keep a written definition of the monitor in the folder that houses all the data for that monitor," says the security officer. "It's stored on our computer, which is linked with the safety officer's computer. That way, we have backup in case one computer goes down." The security officer then describes how he works with his staff to effectively and appropriately collect and utilize data for the monitor.

➡ *At the Office of a Senior Leader.* Finally, the surveyor stops by the office of a senior leader and asks how leadership prioritizes the performance improvement recommendations it receives from throughout the organization. [15] The purpose of this conversation is to see whether the senior leader's description of the process matches the safety officer's.

➡ *Moving Forward.* In closing, the surveyor verifies that EC performance improvement recommendations receive the same level of attention as clinical and administrative recommendations.

At-a-glance
Compliance Strategies

The nature of an organization's performance monitors depends on the type, size, location, and needs of the particular organization. Selection should begin by determining what needs to be measured to illustrate effective management of the EC program. This will prompt the organization to choose meaningful monitors. When identifying possible performance monitors, an organization should consider the following issues:

- Staff knowledge and skills
- Level of staff participation
- Monitoring and inspection activities
- Emergency and incident reporting
- Inspection, maintenance, and testing

Scenario 7-1.
Sample Tracer Questions

The bracketed numbers before each question correlate to questions, observations, and data review described in the sample tracer for Scenario 7-1. You can use the tracer worksheet form in Appendix B to develop a mock tracer (*see* an example of a completed tracer worksheet at the end of this section). The information gained by conducting a mock tracer can help to highlight a good practice and/or determine issues that may require further follow-up.

The Safety Officer

[1] What are the organization's processes for creating performance monitors?

[2] How often are those monitors created?

[3] Why are specific monitors created?

[4] How long have specific monitors been in use?

[5] What do these specific monitors measure?

[6] What methods of data collection are associated with these specific monitors?

[7] What does the organization do with information collected using performance monitors?

[8] How do you use performance monitor data to recommend EC–related improvement activities to organization leadership?

[9] How does leadership prioritize the performance improvement recommendation(s) it receives from throughout the organization?

[10] Do you document what performance improvement projects are selected for implementation during any given year?

Security Manager

[11] How does your department collect data for the performance monitor related to unauthorized after-hours access?

[12] Do you have any documentation on that monitor?

[13] Where do you keep that documentation?

[14] With whom do you share that documentation?

Senior Leader

[15] How does leadership prioritize the performance improvement recommendation(s) it receives from throughout the organization?

Summary

In the following scenario, a surveyor traces how an organization reviews its EC management plans. Within the tracer, the surveyor explores issues relating to these priority focus areas:

- Communication
- Orientation and Training
- Physical Environment
- Quality Improvement Activities

Scenario

As a surveyor looks through an organization's EC management plans, he notes that the plans do not indicate whether they have been recently reviewed. The surveyor decides to trace the organization's process for reviewing its management plans.

(Bracketed numbers correlate to Sample Tracer Questions on page 114.)

➡ *At the Office of the EC Officer.* The surveyor begins the tracer at the office of the EC officer, where he chats with several EC leaders, including the EC officer, the security officer, and the facility manager.

"What is your process for reviewing the EC management plans?" asks the surveyor. [1] "Each year, all the EC leaders get together and evaluate each of the six management plans—safety, security, hazardous materials and waste, fire safety, medical equipment, and utilities," says the EC officer. "During this process, we look at each plan's objectives, scope, performance—how the plan helps reduce risk and keep patients safe. We also look at effectiveness—what went well and what didn't go so well during the year. Basically, we are making sure that the plans do what they set out to do. And if they don't, we work to fix them. To help with this evaluation, we've structured our plans to include sections for objective, scope, performance, and effectiveness. This helps the evaluation process go much more smoothly."

The surveyor then asks how the organization updates the management plans. For example, how does it incorporate any new information or developments that have occurred since the last time plans were evaluated? He probes for details on how the organization ensures that each plan's objectives, performance monitors, and scope definition are still appropriate. [2–3]

The surveyor then presses for information about who participates in the evaluation process and how the organization ensures that it occurs annually. He also asks if the organization documents when the evaluations take place because he noticed that the plans don't reflect that documentation. The EC leaders show the surveyor their annual review report, which does show the date, but they acknowledge that the plans themselves do not include a date. They make a note to include the date at the bottom of the plans in order to document that the plans are current. [4–6]

The surveyor then asks whether the organization compares the annual evaluations against the minutes of its multidisciplinary improvement committee to help identify any unresolved issues and ensure that the minutes support the conclusions of the annual evaluations. [7]

The surveyor also asks what is done with the annual evaluations, including how the EC leaders communicate the results of the evaluation process to organization leadership. [8–9] "We use the annual evaluations as a starting point for further conversation about significant issues affecting the EC," says

At-a-glance
Compliance Strategies

The annual evaluation process should not just inform EC leaders about accomplishments and barriers in the EC. The process should also engender two-way communication between EC leaders and organization leaders, such as senior leaders and board members. Although The Joint Commission does not specify who should receive the annual evaluation, organizations should consider sharing it with senior leadership, boards of directors, department heads, and others in the organization who could benefit from the information. EC leaders can share the evaluation during management meetings, at board meetings, or as a stand-alone memo with a cover sheet. As with a corporate annual report, the annual evaluation of EC management plans should be easy to read and understand. Ideally, it should be in a format that lends itself to presentation, so that content can be quickly and effectively communicated to leadership.

MOCK TRACER TIP

When conducting a mock tracer to reveal how an organization reviews its management plans, remember that no organization is perfect, so the annual evaluation process should not be just a rubber stamp on an organization's EC efforts. The evaluation should realistically identify what the organization did well and what needs to be improved. As a result of the evaluation process, an organization should know which goals and objectives it has and has not met and should be able to identify goals and objectives for the coming year.

the security officer. "Leaders won't read a 50-page analysis, so we create an easy-to-digest document that highlights issues and opens the door for further conversation. Many times, we create a PowerPoint presentation based on the annual evaluations that we can give to senior leaders as well as department leaders."

➡ *At the Office of a Senior Leader.* After speaking with EC leadership, the surveyor stops by the office of a senior leader and asks her about the annual management plan evaluations and inquires if they are easy to read and understand and whether the plans give her a sense of the organization's main EC issues. He also asks what follow-up conversations occur as a result of these evaluations. In this conversation, the surveyor is trying to determine whether the evaluation process meets the needs of senior leadership and promotes open communication about EC issues. [10–13]

➡ *Moving Forward.* The surveyor returns to the office of the EC officer and mentions that the senior leader indicated that the EC evaluations are both thorough and helpful. The surveyor also comments that the senior leader would be open to more regular face-to-face interaction with EC leadership. The EC officer makes a note to connect with the senior leader about this possibility.

Scenario 7-2.
Sample Tracer Questions

The bracketed numbers before each question correlate to questions, observations, and data review described in the sample tracer for Scenario 7-2. You can use the tracer worksheet form in Appendix B to develop a mock tracer (*see* an example of a completed tracer worksheet at the end of this section). The information gained by conducting a mock tracer can help to highlight a good practice and/or determine issues that may require further follow-up.

EC Leaders

[1] Describe the process for reviewing the EC management plans.

[2] How does the organization update the management plans with any new information or developments that have occurred since the last evaluation?

[3] How does the organization ensure that each plan's objectives, performance monitors, and scope definition are still appropriate?

[4] Who participates in the evaluation process?

[5] How does the organization ensure that the evaluation process occurs annually?

[6] Does the organization document the date of evaluations?

[7] Does the organization compare the annual evaluations against the minutes of its multidisciplinary improvement committee?

[8] How do EC leaders communicate the results of the evaluation process to organization leadership?

[9] How do EC leaders use the evaluations as a starting point for further conversation?

Senior Leader

[10] How do you feel about the EC annual management plan evaluations?

[11] Are these evaluations easy to read and understand?

[12] Describe the organization's main EC issues.

[13] What conversations occur about EC issues, based on the annual evaluations?

Sample Tracer Worksheet: Scenario 7-2.

The worksheet below is an example of how organizations can use the sample tracer questions for Scenario 7-2 in a worksheet format during a mock tracer. The bracketed numbers before each question correlate to questions described in the scenario.

A **correct answer** is an appropriate answer that meets the requirements of the organization and other governing bodies. An **incorrect answer** should always include recommendations for follow-up.

Tracer Team Member(s): Jack Schaeffer
Subjects Interviewed: Don Jones, Jacquie Levy, Marion Drake, Annabeth Little
Tracer Topic: EC management plans

Data Record(s): Emergency Operations Plan (EOP); Hazard Vulnerability Analysis (HVA); critique summary
Unit(s) or Department(s): EC officer's office, senior leader's office

Interview Subject: EC Leaders

Questions	Correct Answer	Incorrect Answer	Follow-Up Needed	Comments or Notes
[1] Describe the process for reviewing the EC management plans.	✓			Describes a thorough process for evaluating the plans that involves EC leaders and that occurs annually. The plans are nicely structured to include a section on objectives, scope, performance, and evaluation.
[2] How does the organization update the management plans with any new information or developments that have occurred since the last evaluation?		✓	Should review plans against EC committee meeting minutes to identify new issues. Also, may want to consider using a brief survey that each member of the management plan review team can complete before the evaluation meeting. This could help identify new issues as well.	Although the process for reviewing the plans is good, the process for updating with new info could use some work.

(continued)

Interview Subject: EC Leaders (continued)

Questions	Correct Answer	Incorrect Answer	Follow-Up Needed	Comments or Notes
[3] How does the organization ensure that each plan's objectives, performance monitors, and scope definition are still appropriate?	✓			Good process for double-checking these. EC leaders spend time reviewing these during the evaluation.
[4] Who participates in the evaluation process?		✓	Look at including staff in the process. Discuss this with leaders at the next meeting of the EC committee.	Only EC leaders. May want to consider including frontline EC staff in the discussion, specifically security officers, maintenance managers, and so forth.
[5] How does the organization ensure that the evaluation processes occur annually?	✓			Tickler file reminds EC officer to schedule the meeting. Occurs every year in August.
[6] Does the organization document the date of evaluations?		✓	Adding evaluation date to the bottom of each plan.	Although not required, EC leaders should document the evaluation date on the plan itself to improve communication about when the review occurred.
[7] Does the organization compare the annual evaluations against the minutes of its multidisciplinary improvement committee?		✓	Adding an agenda item to the annual evaluation meeting to review the evaluation in the context of the EC committee meeting minutes.	No, and they should do this to make sure they identify any unresolved issues. Also, this helps link the two documents together and ensures that they don't contradict each other.
[8] How do EC leaders communicate the results of the evaluation process to organization leadership?	✓			Sends report with cover sheet to senior leadership. Does presentation at the board meeting. Shares a copy of the evaluation with department heads (usually using presentation software).

Interview Subject: EC Leaders (continued)				
Questions	**Correct Answer**	**Incorrect Answer**	**Follow-Up Needed**	**Comments or Notes**
[9] How do EC leaders use the evaluations as a starting point for further conversation?		✓	EC leaders and senior leaders should work to set up a meeting following the release of the evaluation report to discuss the highlights of the evaluation in further detail. This will help ensure a more in-depth analysis and also bring senior leaders up to speed on EC issues affecting the organization.	There is a little of this, but the potential for further discussion is great.

Interview Subject: Senior Leader				
Questions	**Correct Answer**	**Incorrect Answer**	**Follow-Up Needed**	**Comments or Notes**
[10–11] How do you feel about the EC annual management plan evaluations? Are they easy to read and understand?	✓			Seems comfortable with the evaluation format. Easy to read and highlights the issues well. Likes the presentation for the board as well.
[12] Describe the organization's main EC issues.		✓	Review the design of the evaluations to make sure they are communicating the level of importance associated with each issue.	Not as familiar with these as she should be. Some of them, including security and HVAC, could be quite problematic for the organization.

(continued)

Interview Subject: Senior Leader (continued)				
Questions	**Correct Answer**	**Incorrect Answer**	**Follow-Up Needed**	**Comments or Notes**
[13] What conversations occur about EC issues, based on the annual evaluations?		✓	Look into creating a follow-up meeting in which senior leaders and EC leaders can further explore EC issues. This may help put EC on the radar screen for performance improvement projects (i.e., the HVAC system).	Again, conversations could be much more in-depth. Right now, there is not a structure for this further follow-up. May want to consider this, so the organization can really stress the importance of EC issues.

Tracer Scenarios for
EMERGENCY MANAGEMENT

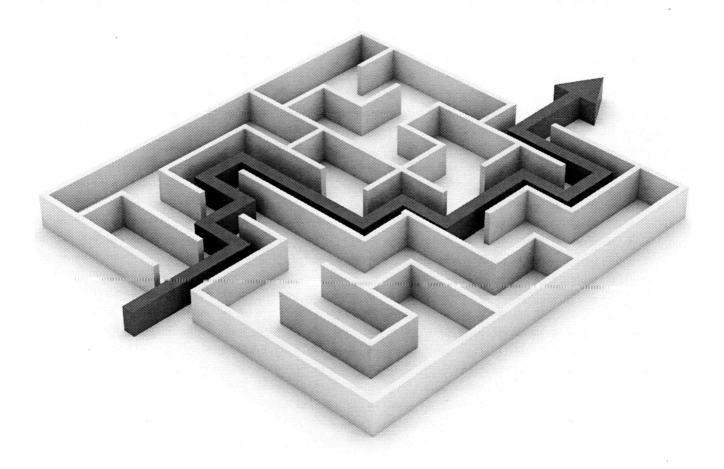

NOTE: No Two Tracers Are the Same

Please keep in mind that each tracer is unique. There is no way to know all of the questions that might be asked or documents that might be reviewed during a tracer—or what all the responses to the questions and documents might be. The possibilities are limitless, depending on the tracer topic and the organization's circumstances. These tracer scenarios and sample questions are provided as educational or training tools for organization staff; they are not scripts for real or mock tracers.

Section Elements

This section includes sample tracers—called scenarios—relevant to emergency management. The section is organized as follows:

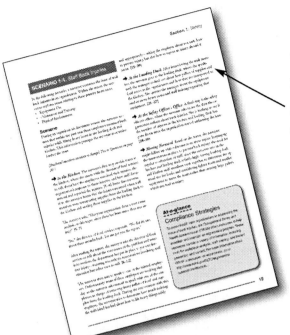

Scenarios: Each scenario presents what might happen when a surveyor conducts a specific type of tracer. The scenarios are presented in an engaging narrative format in which the reader "follows" the surveyor through the tracer scenario. Within the narrative are bracketed numbers that correspond to numbered sample tracer questions following the tracer.

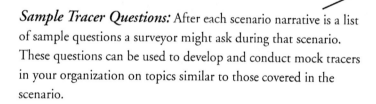

Sample Tracer Questions: After each scenario narrative is a list of sample questions a surveyor might ask during that scenario. These questions can be used to develop and conduct mock tracers in your organization on topics similar to those covered in the scenario.

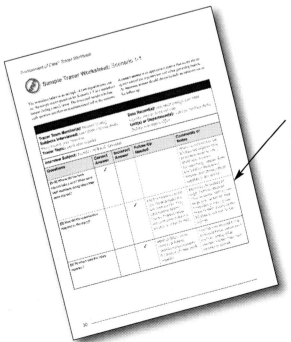

Sample Tracer Worksheet: At the end of the section is a sample worksheet that shows how the sample tracer questions for one select scenario in the section might be used in a worksheet format. The example shows how the worksheet might be completed as part of a tracer for that scenario. A blank form of the worksheet is available in Appendix B.

SCENARIO 8-1. Activating and Operating an Incident Command Center

Summary

In the following scenario, a surveyor traces how an organization activates and operates its incident command center. Within the tracer, the surveyor explores issues relating to these priority focus areas:

- Communication
- Orientation and Training
- Patient Safety
- Physical Environment

Scenario

When reviewing the minutes of an organization's environment of care (EC) committee meetings, a surveyor notes that the organization recently managed an emergency response to a hurricane. Curious about how the organization set up and operated its incident command center during this event, the surveyor decides to trace the topic.

(Bracketed numbers correlate to Sample Tracer Questions on pages 122–123.)

→ *At the Office of the Nursing Supervisor.* The surveyor first speaks with the incident commander of the hurricane response—a nursing supervisor for the organization. The surveyor asks him about his role as incident commander and what that role entails. [1] She also asks him about any training he received on how to be an incident commander and whether he feels that training helped him during the hurricane. The surveyor probes for further information on why the organization chose the nursing supervisor to be the incident commander, what he does to prepare for an incident, and whether there is someone else who can take his place if he is unavailable. [2–5] In this conversation, the surveyor is trying to assess how comfortable the nursing supervisor is with his role and whether he is adequately prepared for all that the role entails.

After this conversation, the surveyor asks to see where the incident command center is located. [6] The nursing supervisor takes her to the primary location, explaining that the organization also has a secondary location to use in the event that the primary location becomes inaccessible during an emergency. "We also have a process in place for a virtual command center," says the nursing supervisor. "We use this during pro-

longed emergencies that spread across the facility, such as during high-census flu seasons." [7–9]

→ *At the Incident Command Center.* At the incident command center, the surveyor presses the nursing supervisor for information about how the command center is activated, set up, and equipped. She asks if the organization uses an incident command system, such as the National Incident Management System (NIMS) or the Hospital Incident Command System (HICS). She then asks the nursing supervisor to describe briefly how the organization's system of choice works. [11–13]

Following this discussion, the surveyor examines the incident command center, opening cabinets and looking in closets. During this tour, she asks detailed questions about the number of emergency power outlets in the area and whether all systems in the area are tied to emergency power. [14–15]

She also asks about emergency supplies: "What types of emergency supplies does the organization keep in this area?" [16] "We have a lot in here—vests—these help staff, patients, and visitors know who is on the incident command team—clipboards, flashlights, PPE [personal protective equipment], two-way radios, marking pens, and more," says the nursing supervisor. "Along

At-a-glance
Compliance Strategies

An incident command system helps an organization identify who is in charge during an emergency—the incident commander—and the individuals who will carry out the objectives of the individual in charge. It establishes a chain of communication and accountability to support situational awareness, efficient decision making, and ongoing feedback on response actions. Everyone in an organization should understand the basic principles of the incident command system and how it applies during an emergency. An incident command system should be adjustable in size and scope so that it can be adapted to emergencies of all types and magnitudes, reflecting an all-hazards approach. Building in this kind of flexibility facilitates decision making at the time of an incident rather than attempting to plan every potential detail of a dynamic and evolving event ahead of time.

with one of my colleagues, I went through this area after the hurricane and restocked it in preparation for the next event."

The surveyor asks about the last emergency response, querying whether the supplies present were adequate or whether something was missing. She also probes for more details about special equipment. [17–18]

The surveyor then asks about the alternative location for the incident command center, why the organization chose that location, and whether the organization has ever used it.

"Has the organization ever done an emergency management drill using the alternative location?" says the surveyor. [10] "No, we've always used this location," says the nursing supervisor. "But that's a really good idea. I will suggest that at our next EM [emergency management] committee meeting."

➡ *Community Interaction.* Pursuing a slightly different topic, the surveyor asks the nursing supervisor how the incident command center connects to community responders and whether the organization has an interactive relationship with those community responders. She asks about this relationship and how often the organization and emergency responders get together to talk about emergency response. [19–21]

➡ *Incident Command Team Members.* Next, the surveyor moves on to questions about the incident command team members. She asks the nursing supervisor who is on the team and what their different roles are. [22–23]

"Which team members are stationed in the command center during an emergency?" asks the surveyor. [24] "Certainly me because I have primary responsibility for management and direction of the event response," says the nursing supervisor. "Also, our communications person, safety officer, and security officer are stationed here. Depending on the size of the emergency, we might add some clerical staff as well. During the hurricane, we had two clerical people here at all times."

Finally, the surveyor asks about reporting structures for the team during an emergency. The nursing supervisor shows her the incident command system's organizational chart, which clearly defines the roles of the incident command team and the duties and responsibilities associated with those roles. The surveyor asks whether the organization shares this chart with all staff members, so they can be clear about who they report to during an emergency. [25–26]

➡ *On a Patient Care Unit.* After talking with the nursing supervisor, the surveyor goes to a nearby patient care unit, where she talks to a staff person. The surveyor asks the staff person if he knows where the incident command center is and who works there. The surveyor asks who the staff person reported to during the hurricane response and whether he was clear on the reporting structure before the start of the hurricane. The surveyor also asks the staff member to describe his responsibilities during the emergency response and whether he felt comfortable with those responsibilities. [27–32]

➡ *Moving Forward.* Based on the tracer, the surveyor might follow up with a discussion on these topics with the nursing supervisor: providing additional training and education to frontline staff about the incident command system, including who is in charge during an emergency and where the incident command center—and alternative incident command center—is located, and providing further training on staff responsibilities during an emergency to reinforce the importance of everyone's role.

MOCK TRACER TIP

When performing a mock tracer on an organization's incident command center, check whether the primary and secondary sites for the center are on emergency backup power. During an emergency is not the time to discover that the command center is dependent on a fully functioning electrical system. This can cost the organization critical time as incident team members search for ways to reestablish power to the area.

Scenario 8-1. Sample Tracer Questions

The bracketed numbers before each question correlate to questions, observations, and data review described in the sample tracer for Scenario 8-1. You can use the tracer worksheet form in Appendix B to develop a mock tracer (*see* an example of a completed tracer worksheet at the end of this section). The information gained by conducting a mock tracer can help to highlight a good practice and/or determine issues that may require further follow-up.

Nursing Supervisor (Incident Commander)

[1] Describe your role as incident commander.

[2] What training have you received about how to be an incident commander?

[3] Did that training help you during the recent emergency response?

[4] Why did the organization choose you to be the incident commander? Is there a backup person in case you are unavailable?

[5] What do you do to prepare for an incident?

[6] Show me the incident command center.

[7] Why did the organization choose this location for the command center?

[8] Does the organization have a secondary location?

[9] Why did the organization choose that location?

[10] Has the organization ever done an emergency management drill using the alternative location?

[11] How does the organization activate the incident command center? set it up? equip it?

[12] Does the organization use an incident command system, such as NIMS or HICS?

[13] Describe the incident command system the organization uses.

[14] How many emergency power outlets does this area have?

[15] Are all systems in the area tied to emergency power?

[16] What types of emergency supplies does the organization keep in this area?

[17] During the last emergency response, were the number and types of supplies adequate? Was anything missing?

[18] What types of equipment does the organization keep here?

[19] How does the incident command center connect to community responders?

[20] Does this organization have an interactive relationship with community responders?

[21] How often do people from the organization and emergency responders get together to talk about emergency response?

[22] Who is on the incident command team?

[23] What are the roles of the different team members?

[24] Which team members are stationed in the command center during an emergency?

[25] What are the reporting structures for the incident command system?

[26] How does the organization communicate with staff about those reporting structures?

Patient Care Unit Staff Member

[27] Where is the incident command center?

[28] Who works there?

[29] Who did you report to during the last emergency response event?

[30] Did you know you would report to that person before the event?

[31] What were your responsibilities during the last emergency response?

[32] Were you comfortable with those responsibilities?

SCENARIO 8-2. Retracing an Emergency Response

Summary

In the following scenario, a surveyor traces an organization's response to an emergency involving decontamination. Within the tracer, the surveyor explores issues relating to these priority focus areas:

- Communication
- Equipment Use
- Orientation and Training
- Patient Safety
- Physical Environment

Scenario

During an organization's EM session, a surveyor learns that the organization recently experienced an emergency involving a woman who arrived at the hospital after having contact with an explosive device containing an unknown substance. This emergency necessitated the use of the hospital's decontamination facilities. Curious about the organization's response to the incident, the surveyor decides to trace what happened.

(Bracketed numbers correlate to Sample Tracer Questions on pages 125–126.)

➜ *At the EC Office.* First, the surveyor sits down with the organization's EM officer to talk about the event. "Could you describe how the event started?" asks the surveyor. [1] "Sure," says the EM officer. "Basically, a young woman in our community found a homemade explosive device in her driveway, and it blew up in her face. Emergency medical services (EMS) responded to the scene. On the way to the hospital, EMS called ahead to inform our staff that the incoming victim had been exposed to an unknown oily chemical substance. Together, the risk manager, chief nursing officer, and I determined that it was time to activate our incident command system and emergency response effort."

"What happened next?" prompts the surveyor. "Based on our conversations with the EMS team, we were reasonably certain that the substance was not an airborne contaminant because the only people who had reactions were those who had physical contact with it," says the EM officer. "To be as safe as possible, though, we taped off a large section of the ED [emergency department] and parking lot. We thought we had the situation under control, but we missed taping off one of the internal doors—and a staff member accidentally walked through it, from the decon area, around the patient, and into the main area of the ED. So, we went into lockdown mode and called a code yellow—emergency disaster."

After the EM officer initially describes the incident, the surveyor asks for further details. He first asks how the organization locked down the ED. He then asks how EMS addressed ventilation issues associated with the ED. He also asks how the organization worked with its community partners during the event. He is trying to discover how the organization addressed the six critical areas of EM—communication, resources and assets, safety and security, staff responsibilities, utilities management, and patient support—during the event. [2–5]

Next, the surveyor probes for information on how the organization kept patients and staff in the locked-down ED calm and comfortable. The surveyor and the EM officer discuss how the organization shared information with patients and staff, including how it used cell phones, pagers, and two-way radios to do this. [6–8]

➜ *Establishing the Need for Decontamination.* The surveyor asks how the organization determined that it needed to decontaminate patients and visitors.

"How did the organization identify the unknown chemical substance?" asks the surveyor. [9] "We sent a sample of the material

MOCK TRACER TIP

One way to expand the depth of an emergency management mock tracer is to ask a series of "what if" questions. What if, during this emergency, the power went out? What if the individual came in to the hospital at 3 A.M. instead of during the regular business day? What if the organization wasn't able to find out what the chemical substance was for 36 hours? These types of questions can help further drill down into the organization's preparedness efforts and expose areas of risk.

At-a-glance
Compliance Strategies

When planning for decontamination activities, organizations should coordinate with their community and determine what resources the fire department or emergency managers can provide. Organizations with a military facility located close by should consider establishing a relationship with that facility as it may be better equipped than the health care facility to provide radioactive, biological, and chemical isolation and decontamination.

In addition, organizations should consider consulting with their local emergency planning committee (LEPC). Every community must have an LEPC, as mandated by the Occupational Safety and Health Administration (OSHA). The LEPC has information about hazardous chemicals in the area and knows what companies and organizations use these chemicals. Because of the wealth of information it must collect to meet federal requirements, the LEPC can be a valuable—and largely untapped—resource for health care organizations on how to address individuals who come in contact with hazardous chemicals.

off site for testing," says the EM officer. "It took several hours, but the laboratory finally let us know that the material was not an airborne contaminant. However, the lab did suggest having all exposed individuals go through decontamination."

Based on this answer, the surveyor spends some time asking how the hospital set up decontamination facilities and what was involved with that. He asks whether the decontamination effort went according to plan. He also asks for information on the role of the fire department in decontamination procedures. [10–13]

The surveyor then asks how the organization dealt with new patients arriving at the ED during the time of the lockdown. The surveyor and the EM officer discuss where those patients were sent in the building and how they were triaged. [14–15]

The surveyor follows up this conversation by asking what happened after the lockdown was lifted, specifically probing for information about how the organization resumed normal operations. [16–18]

➡ *In the ED.* After speaking with the EM officer, the surveyor goes to the ED, where he asks to speak with someone who was locked in during the event. He is introduced to a nurse who tells him about the lockdown and her perspective on it. [22] The surveyor presses for information on how the organization kept things calm in the ED and communicated with everyone there. He also asks about her role in the response and whether she felt she was prepared for the role. Then he asks about the decontamination process and how that went. Finally, he asks her if there was anything about the response that could have been done differently. [23–28]

➡ *Moving Forward.* The surveyor returns to the EM officer's office and asks whether the organization performed an analysis of the emergency response and identified areas for improvement. The surveyor and the EM officer discuss what the organization learned and how it's using that information to plan for and improve performance during the next emergency. [19–21].

Scenario 8-2.
Sample Tracer Questions

The bracketed numbers before each question correlate to questions, observations, and data review described in the sample tracer for Scenario 8-2. You can use the tracer worksheet form in Appendix B to develop a mock tracer (*see* an example of a completed tracer worksheet at the end of this section). The information gained by conducting a mock tracer can help to highlight a good practice and/or determine issues that may require further follow-up.

EM Officer

[1] Describe how the event unfolded.

[2] How did the organization lock down the ED?

[3] How did the organization address potential ventilation issues?

[4] How did the organization work with its community partners during the event?

[5] How did the organization address the six critical areas of EM during the event?

[6] How did the organization keep patients and staff in the locked-down ED calm and comfortable?

[7] How did the organization share information with patients and staff?

[8] Did the organization use cell phones, pagers, and two-way radios to share information among patients and staff? If so, how did those work?

[9] How did the organization identify the unknown chemical substance?

[10] How did the hospital set up decontamination facilities?

[11] Did the decontamination effort go according to plan?

[12] Were there any glitches in the process?

[13] What was the role of the fire department in the decontamination procedures?

[14] How did the organization deal with new patients arriving at the ED during the time of the lockdown?

[15] Where were those patients sent in the building, and how were they triaged?

[16] How did the organization determine when to lift the lockdown?

(continued)

Scenario 8-2.
Sample Tracer Questions (continued)

[17] What happened after the lockdown was lifted?

[18] How did the organization resume normal operations?

[19] Did the organization perform an analysis of the emergency response?

[20] What areas of improvement did the organization identify?

[21] How did the organization respond to this information?

Nurse in the ED

[22] Describe the lockdown and what it was like.

[23] How did the organization keep things calm during the lockdown?

[24] How did the organization communicate with you?

[25] What was your role during the emergency response?

[26] Did you feel you were prepared for the role?

[27] How did the decontamination process go?

[28] Was there anything about the response that could have been done differently?

SCENARIO 8-3. Planning for an Emergency

Summary

In the following scenario, a surveyor traces an organization's administrative activities associated with preparing for an emergency. Within the tracer, the surveyor explores issues relating to these priority focus areas:

- Communication
- Orientation and Training
- Patient Safety
- Physical Environment

Scenario

As a surveyor reviews an organization's EM documents, he wonders if the organization has a detailed and interdisciplinary process for creating a hazard vulnerability analysis (HVA) and an Emergency Operations Plan (EOP). The surveyor decides to further explore how the organization develops these tools and ensures an integrated emergency response.

(Bracketed numbers correlate to Sample Tracer Questions on page 128.)

→ *At the Office of Safety Officer.* The surveyor starts the tracer by asking the safety officer about the HVA.

"How did the organization create its HVA?" asks the surveyor. [1–3] "We use a multidisciplinary process, which includes our EC staff, organization leaders, nurses, physicians, and support staff," says the safety officer. "We actually have an HVA committee that convenes once a year to review the document and make changes as necessary. Members of our EC committee sit on the HVA committee, but there are other people who participate as well." The safety officer goes on to explain how senior leadership is involved in the HVA process, along with community partners, such as members of the local fire department, police department, and other emergency preparedness personnel.

"When this HVA planning team meets, how does it conduct the HVA?" asks the surveyor. "Well, the first time we did this, we made a list of all possible disasters that could affect our organization," says the safety officer. "Then we ranked the most likely and critical emergencies as well as the emergencies for which we are well prepared. This helped us focus our efforts on the most critical areas of risk. Now when we meet, we do an abbreviated version of this process to ensure that we are addressing the most important risks. Some disasters have remained on the HVA every year, and others have fallen off or been added, depending on their perceived importance. Probably our top three emergencies are an ice/snow storm that shuts down power, a chemical spill at the nearby plastics plant, and a multivehicle accident on one of the four highways that pass within 15 miles of our organization." [4]

The surveyor follows up this answer with a few more questions about the HVA, including how it is documented, how it is used to define mitigation and preparedness activities, and how its content and recommendations are coordinated with the community. [5–7]

→ *Review of the EOP.* Next, the surveyor reviews the organization's EOP. As he is looking through the plan, he asks the safety officer to explain how organization leadership, including medical staff, participate in plan development. [8] He then probes for details about what the organization would do if it had a prolonged absence of community support during an emergency. [9] In this conversation, he is trying to determine whether the organization has considered how long it can provide safe patient care and how patients will have their care needs met for up to 96 hours. He specifically asks the safety officer to talk about this scenario as it relates to the top three emergencies on the organization's HVA.

The surveyor then asks how the organization addresses the six critical areas of EM—communication, resources and assets, safety and security, staff responsibilities, utilities management, and patient support—and supports an all-hazards approach in the EOP. He asks the safety officer to give an example of how

the organization would address each of the six critical areas during the top three emergencies discussed in the HVA. [10]

The surveyor also asks to see the organization's written inventory of resources and assets that may be needed during an emergency, looking to see if this organization lists PPE, water, fuel, and medical, surgical, and medication-related items.

After this, the surveyor asks the safety officer to describe the processes used to initiate and terminate response and recovery efforts, including what circumstances would warrant these efforts and who has the authority to initiate them. He also asks about the organization's alternative care sites, how they were chosen, in what situations they would be used, and whether a drill has been done at one of these sites. [11–17]

➡ *On a Patient Care Unit.* After speaking with the safety officer, the surveyor visits a patient care unit and asks to speak with a staff member. He asks the staff member about the top emergencies the organization might face and whether she feels the organization is prepared for those emergencies. He asks her to describe some of the things the organization has done to prepare for emergencies, as well as what her role would be in an emergency situation and whether she is comfortable with that role. [18–22] He is trying to determine whether frontline staff understand the organization's emergency planning documents. He also wants to confirm that the organization addresses the concerns staff members have about potential emergencies and how the organization would respond to these concerns.

At-a-glance
Compliance Strategies

A critical component of the EOP is a description of how the organization will sustain itself during an emergency. Specifically, the EOP must be robust enough to help guide organizational decision making for emergencies that may be of long duration—96 hours—when the organization cannot be supported by its local community.

There are many issues to consider when planning for sustainability, from the supply of medications to treat patients to the amount of fuel needed to power the emergency generators. An organization should take a proactive look at its resources and determine what type of services it can and cannot provide at different points during the 96 hours.

An organization may opt to remain open for less than 96 hours and choose to curtail services or evacuate instead—for example, after 48 hours. However, evacuation is not always possible during an escalating emergency, and sometimes an organization is unable to evacuate but still needs to provide services to its patients. An organization should write its EOP according to various possible scenarios.

It is also important to share any information about sustainability with community partners: They need to understand what a health care organization can and cannot do during an emergency. This allows everyone to plan accordingly and ensures a coordinated and effective response.

MOCK TRACER TIP

When conducting a mock tracer that focuses on an organization's emergency planning efforts, it is critical to determine how the organization coordinates its plans with the community. The standards stress the need for this coordination, specifically when creating the HVA and EOP. Drilling down and discovering how the organization communicates with the community and involves it in the planning process can help ensure compliance with this portion of the standards. As part of this exploration, speak to community partners, if possible—such as other hospitals or health care organizations, EMS, police, and the health department—and gain their perspective on how the organization coordinates emergency preparedness.

➡ *Moving Forward.* Based on the tracer, the surveyor might follow up with a discussion with the safety officer on continuing the efforts to involve the community in emergency planning efforts—including those related to the HVA and EOP. Most large-scale emergencies affect not only the hospital but also the community, and so proactive plans that take into consideration the needs and resources of the community will more likely help the organization navigate a successful response.

Scenario 8-3.
Sample Tracer Questions

The bracketed numbers before each question correlate to questions, observations, and data review described in the sample tracer for Scenario 8-3. You can use the tracer worksheet form in Appendix B to develop a mock tracer (*see* an example of a completed tracer worksheet at the end of this section). The information gained by conducting a mock tracer can help to highlight a good practice and/or determine issues that may require further follow-up.

Safety Officer in Charge of EM

[1] How does the organization create its HVA?

[2] How does the organization involve senior leadership in the process?

[3] How does the organization involve community partners in the process?

[4] What are the organization's top three emergencies?

[5] How is the HVA process documented?

[6] How is the HVA used to define mitigation and preparedness activities?

[7] How are the contents and recommendations in the HVA coordinated with the community?

[8] How does organization leadership, including medical staff, participate in developing the EOP?

[9] What would the organization do if it had a 96-hour absence of community support during an emergency? Talk about this scenario as it relates to the organization's top three emergencies.

[10] How does the organization address the six critical areas of EM? Give an example of how the organization would address each of these areas during the top three emergencies discussed in the HVA.

[11] Describe the processes used to initiate and terminate response and recovery efforts.

[12] What circumstances would warrant these efforts?

[13] Who has the authority to initiate these efforts?

[14] Describe the organization's alternative care sites.

[15] How were these sites chosen?

[16] In what situations would these sites would be used?

[17] Has the organization ever done a drill using an alternative care site?

Patient Care Unit Staff Member

[18] What do you think are the top emergencies the organization might face?

[19] Do you think the organization is prepared to respond to those emergencies?

[20] Describe some of the things the organization has done to prepare for emergencies.

[21] What would be your role in an emergency situation?

[22] Are you comfortable with that role?

SCENARIO 8-4. Disaster Privileging

Summary

In the following scenario, a surveyor traces an organization's processes for granting privileges in a disaster. Within the tracer, the surveyor explores issues relating to these priority focus areas:

- Communication
- Credentialed Practitioners
- Orientation and Training
- Patient Safety

Scenario

As a surveyor reviews an organization's EM documents, she stops to read the organization's policy on granting disaster privileges to volunteer licensed independent practitioners and other volunteer practitioners. The surveyor wants to determine whether the organization understands and can effectively carry out its policy during an emergency. Consequently, she decides to trace the disaster privileging process.

(Bracketed numbers correlate to Sample Tracer Questions on page 130.)

➔ *The Office of the Chief of Medicine.* The surveyor first sits down with the chief of medicine and asks who in the organization is responsible for granting disaster privileges to volunteer licensed independent practitioners and other volunteer practitioners. She also asks how and where the organization documents this responsibility. [1–2] The chief of medicine explains, "We outline in the medical staff bylaws who is responsible for granting disaster privileges. For our organization, that is either me or, if I am not present, whoever is acting as the chief of medicine during the emergency."

The surveyor then asks the chief of medicine to outline how the process of granting disaster privileges works, including when the organization can grant disaster privileges; to whom it can grant such privileges; how it verifies licensure, certification, or registration required to practice a profession; and how it ensures oversight of the care, treatment, and services provided by the privileged volunteer. [3–6]

"How does the organization distinguish volunteer licensed independent practitioners from other licensed independent practitioners?" asks the surveyor. [7] "We have special orange badges that the volunteers wear," says the chief of medicine. "These have a designated place on them to write the person's name, profession, and privileging status. We keep blank badges in the incident command center for use during an emergency."

The surveyor then asks what types of information the organization is required to get before the privileged volunteer can begin treating patients, such as a valid driver's license, an identification card for another health care organization that identifies professional designation, or a confirmation by a currently privileged licensed independent practitioner. [8]

➔ *Reviewing Documentation on Performance Assessment.* The surveyor asks to see and review documentation from the organization's most recent disaster response during which it was required to grant disaster privileges to volunteer practitioners. During this review, she asks how the organization assesses performance and determines whether to continue granting disaster privileges to an individual. The surveyor and chief of medicine talk not only about the logistics involved in assessing performance but also about who is in charge of the effort. [9–10]

Finally, the surveyor asks about how the organization obtains primary source verification of licensure and when that happens. She specifically probes for information about what the organization does when it is not possible to obtain primary source verification within 72 hours. [11–13]

➔ *On a Patient Care Unit.* The surveyor stops by a patient care unit and talks with a physician on duty. The surveyor asks the physician if she knows how the organization grants disaster privileges to volunteer licensed independent practitioners and other volunteer practitioners. [14] The surveyor does not expect the physician to know every detail of the process but to have a general understanding of it. She asks the physician about any experience she has working with a privileged volunteer licensed independent practitioner during an emergency. The surveyor specifically probes for details on how the volunteer's performance was monitored and how the physician identified that the volunteer was appropriately privileged. The goal of this conversation is to see if the organization's practices match its policies. [15–17]

➔ *Moving Forward.* Based on the tracer, the surveyor might follow up with a discussion about including the disaster privileging process in the organization's next EM exercise. The nuances of disaster privileging can be challenging and practicing how this process would work during a disaster could be very beneficial.

At-a-glance
Compliance Strategies

A number of state and federal systems are engaged in pre-event verification of qualifications for volunteer licensed independent practitioners. Such a system can help facilitate the assigning of disaster privileges during emergencies. Examples include the Emergency System for Advance Registration of Volunteer Health Professionals (ESAR-VHP), created by the Health Resources and Services Administration (HRSA), and the Medical Reserve Corps (MRC). ESAR-VHP allows for the advance registration and credentialing of health care professionals needed to meet increased patient/victim care and increased surge capacity in a health care organization. MRC units are comprised of locally based medical and public health volunteers.

> ## MOCK TRACER TIP
>
> To gain a different perspective on disaster privileging, a surveyor participating in a mock tracer on this topic should talk to a volunteer licensed independent practitioner who has gone through the volunteer privileging process. This discussion might help identify weaknesses in the system that may not be apparent by just reviewing policies and talking with the full-time medical staff.

Scenario 8-4.
Sample Tracer Questions

The bracketed numbers before each question correlate to questions, observations, and data review described in the sample tracer for Scenario 8-4. You can use the tracer worksheet form in Appendix B to develop a mock tracer (*see* an example of a completed tracer worksheet at the end of this section). The information gained by conducting a mock tracer can help to highlight a good practice and/or determine issues that may require further follow-up.

Chief of Medicine

[1] Who is responsible for granting disaster privileges to volunteer licensed independent practitioners and other volunteer practitioners?

[2] How does the organization document this responsibility, and where does it document it?

[3] When can the organization grant disaster privileges?

[4] To whom can it grant such privileges?

[5] How does the organization verify licensure, certification, or registration required to practice a profession?

[6] How does the organization ensure oversight of the care, treatment, and services provided by a privileged volunteer?

[7] How does the organization distinguish volunteer licensed independent practitioners from other licensed independent practitioners?

[8] What types of information is the organization required to get before the privileged volunteer can begin treating patients?

[9] How does the organization assess performance and determine whether to continue granting disaster privileges to an individual?

[10] Who is in charge of making this determination?

[11] How does the organization obtain primary source verification of licensure?

[12] When does this happen?

[13] What would the organization do if it could not obtain primary source verification within 72 hours?

Physician on a Patient Care Unit

[14] Do you know how the organization grants disaster privileges to volunteer licensed independent practitioners and other volunteer practitioners?

[15] Have you ever worked with a privileged volunteer licensed independent practitioner during an emergency? If so, how did the experience go?

[16] How was the volunteer's performance monitored?

[17] How did you recognize this person's privileging status?

Sample Tracer Worksheet: Scenario 8-3.

The worksheet below is an example of how organizations can use the sample tracer questions for Scenario 8-3 in a worksheet format during a mock tracer. The bracketed numbers before each question correlate to questions described in the scenario.

A **correct answer** is an appropriate answer that meets the requirements of the organization and other governing bodies. An **incorrect answer** should always include recommendations for follow-up.

Tracer Team Member(s): Marcus Doyle
Subjects Interviewed: Filipe Jones, Belinda Burke
Tracer Topic: Planning for an Emergency

Data Record(s): Emergency Operations Plan (EOP); Hazard Vulnerability Analysis (HVA); critique summary
Unit(s) or Department(s): Safety officer's office, patient care unit 14B

Interview Subject: Safety Officer in Charge of EM

Questions	Correct Answer	Incorrect Answer	Follow-Up Needed	Comments or Notes
[1] How does the organization create its HVA?	✓			Describes a multidisciplinary process that involves many different departments, including EC, medical staff, nursing, and support staff.
[2] How does the organization involve senior leadership in the process?		✓	Work on improving senior leadership involvement. Maybe do a presentation on the importance of the emergency planning process and what happens when it's not thorough.	Has some senior leadership involvement but could have a lot more. Senior leaders should not only be involved in creating the plan but also using the plan to improve EM response.
[3] How does the organization involve community partners in the process?		✓	Need to work on improving the interactive component of this process. Maybe the fire and police chief can sit on the HVA committee?	The organization has some involvement of the community but could involve them a lot more. For example, there is no representative of the community on the HVA committee, so the organization just presents the completed HVA to the police and fire departments. This isn't overly interactive.

(continued)

Interview Subject: *Safety Officer in Charge of EM (continued)*

Questions	Correct Answer	Incorrect Answer	Follow-Up Needed	Comments or Notes
[4] What are the organization's top three emergencies?	✓			Able to describe these and why they are the organization's top three. Outlines a comprehensive, risk-driven process for conducting the HVA.
[5, 7] How is the HVA process documented? How are the contents and recommendations in the HVA coordinated with the community?		✓	Need to encourage a more interactive discussion about HVA results with the community. Perhaps bring different community partners together for a biannual meeting to discuss the HVA and the EM risks the community and organization face.	Has a written summary of the HVA process, including a description of the organization's top disasters. This is included in the organization's EOP. This is all in order. However, to communicate with the community, the organization just sends a copy of the document to the community responders. Should work on having a more interactive discussion.
[6] How is the HVA used to define mitigation and preparedness activities?	✓			Able to show how the HVA affects mitigation and preparedness. Organization does a good job prioritizing its EM work based on the HVA.
[8] How does organization leadership, including medical staff, participate in developing the EOP?	✓			Much better at involving leadership, including medical staff, in EOP creation. Have a multidisciplinary team that creates the EOP, and senior leadership and medical staff play a prominent role on this team. Should use this process as an example for HVA.

Interview Subject:	Safety Officer in Charge of EM (continued)			
Questions	**Correct Answer**	**Incorrect Answer**	**Follow-Up Needed**	**Comments or Notes**
[9] What would the organization do if it had a 96-hour absence of community support during an emergency? Talk about this scenario as it relates to the organization's top three emergencies.		✓	Perhaps create a small committee to really dig deep on this issue. Could investigate using a dashboard to monitor resources and supplies and help establish a cutoff point for patient care.	Organization hasn't given this as much thought as it should. Thinks it can just plow through. The organization needs to spend some time really looking at resources and supplies and when it will make the cutoff to evacuate and terminate services.
[10] How does the organization address the six critical areas of EM? Give an example of how the organization would address each of these areas during the top three emergencies discussed in the HVA.	✓			Able to do this really well. Can tell this is where the organization is focusing its efforts. Could do better with community involvement and a sustained response, but overall very good work.
[11– 13] Describe the processes used to initiate and terminate response and recovery efforts. What circumstances would warrant these efforts? Who has the authority to initiate them?	✓			Can describe processes for initiating and terminating response and recovery. Names people in charge of these efforts and what types of events warrant this activity.
[14–17] Describe the organization's alternative care sites. How were they chosen? In what situations would they be used? Has the organization ever done a drill using an alternative site?		✓	Need to review these sites and why they were chosen. Maybe need to visit the sites? Maybe another site is better? Also, should consider performing an EM drill using one of the sites to identify strengths and weaknesses.	Although the safety officer can name alternative sites, he isn't too familiar with why those sites were chosen, when they should be used, what the advantages/disadvantages of the sites are, etc. Sites chosen 5 years ago. Safety officer started 3 years ago. Not sure the organization has reviewed the sites since then.

(continued)

Interview Subject: Patient Care Unit Staff Member

Questions	Correct Answer	Incorrect Answer	Follow-Up Needed	Comments or Notes
[18–20] What do you think are the top emergencies the organization might face? Do you think the organization is prepared to respond to those emergencies? Describe some of the things the organization has done to prepare for emergencies.		✓	Although many of the staff member's comments are positive, the organization should follow up about emergencies she lists as concerns and see if adding them to the HVA makes sense. Also should look at what the organization is doing to help family of staff during an emergency. If staff members' family needs are met, they are more likely to show up to help in an emergency and focus on their jobs while at the organization.	Describes similar emergencies as the HVA, but also adds some other ones not found on the HVA—terrorist event, H1N1-type infection, and infant abduction. Has the organization considered these? Why are they not on the list? Nurse seems comfortable with the organization's level of preparation. Gives the impression that the organization has her back and would work with her to navigate an emergency successfully. Does express concern about what would happen to her family during an emergency if she were working. Has an elderly mother living with her and is afraid of what would happen if she left her mother to go to work.
[21–22] What would be your role in an emergency situation? Are you comfortable with that role?	✓			Can describe her role and seems very comfortable with it. Received training on her role and practiced it during a recent drill.

Tracer Scenarios for
LIFE SAFETY

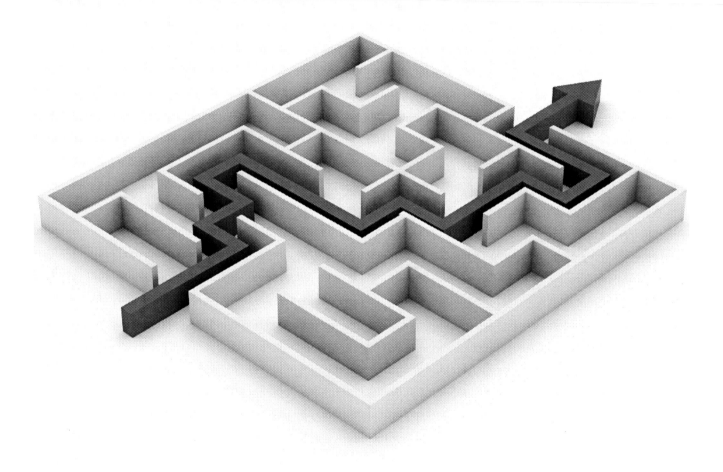

NOTE: No Two Tracers Are the Same

Please keep in mind that each tracer is unique. There is no way to know all of the questions that might be asked or documents that might be reviewed during a tracer—or what all the responses to the questions and documents might be. The possibilities are limitless, depending on the tracer topic and the organization's circumstances. These tracer scenarios and sample questions are provided as educational or training tools for organization staff; they are not scripts for real or mock tracers.

Section Elements

This section includes sample tracers—called scenarios—relevant to life safety. The section is organized as follows:

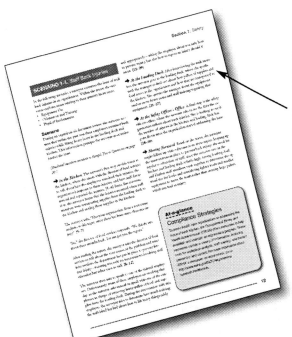

Scenarios: Each scenario presents what might happen when a surveyor conducts a specific type of tracer. The scenarios are presented in an engaging narrative format in which the reader "follows" the surveyor through the tracer scenario. Within the narrative are bracketed numbers that correspond to numbered sample tracer questions following the tracer.

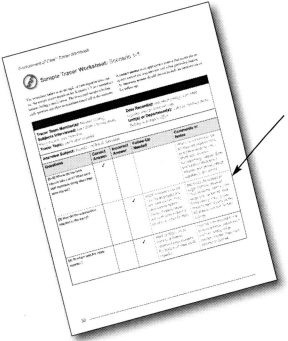

Sample Tracer Questions: After each scenario narrative is a list of sample questions a surveyor might ask during that scenario. These questions can be used to develop and conduct mock tracers in your organization on topics similar to those covered in the scenario.

Sample Tracer Worksheet: At the end of the section is a sample worksheet that shows how the sample tracer questions for one select scenario in the section might be used in a worksheet format. The example shows how the worksheet might be completed as part of a tracer for that scenario. A blank form of the worksheet is available in Appendix B.

SCENARIO 9-1. Touring a Construction Project

Summary

In the following scenario, a surveyor traces how an organization maintains life safety during a construction project. Within the tracer, the surveyor explores issues relating to these priority focus areas:

- Communication
- Orientation and Training
- Patient Safety
- Physical Environment

Scenario

A health care organization is undergoing a construction project on the eastern wing of the building. The project has been under way for about three months and will be completed in about six more months. During the survey, the surveyor decides to trace how the organization maintains life safety during this construction process.

(Bracketed numbers correlate to Sample Tracer Questions on page 139.)

➡ *At the Office of the Facility Manager.* First, the surveyor goes to the office of the facility manager, who is the organization liaison for the construction project. He asks this individual some initial questions about the project, including when it started, how long it is expected to continue, and whether the organization has experienced any problems in the project that could threaten the safety of patients, staff, and visitors. [1–2]

"Do you have a 'no smoking' policy for the area?" asks the surveyor. "And if you do, how do you enforce that policy?" [3–4] "We do not allow anyone to smoke in the construction area, just like we don't allow anyone to smoke anywhere in the building," says the facility manager. "To make sure that construction workers don't smoke, we provided some up-front training on why we have the policy and what the risks are in smoking around the construction site. Each construction worker had to sign an agreement saying he or she would not smoke in the area. We also hung posters throughout the site, reminding people not to smoke. As part of my daily tour of the construction site, I look for people smoking or evidence of people smoking. If I find some, I speak to the general contractor right away, and we address that with the individuals involved."

The surveyor then asks about other training and orientation the organization offers to construction workers. The surveyor and facility manager talk about a variety of education topics, including appropriate paths of travel, required interim life safety measures (ILSM), infection control, removal of dust, proper debris removal, and what to do in case of a fire. The facility manager describes how the organization works with the construction company to provide education and ensure that all workers on the project understand the information taught. [5–8]

The surveyor next addresses the issue of building exits. "Are any building exits compromised by the construction?" asks the

At-a-glance

Compliance Strategies

A general contractor on a health care organization construction project should have health care experience; however, not all construction workers are familiar with the unique issues associated with a health care construction project. For example, a utility shutdown must be carefully planned and coordinated in a health care facility. Workers can't just cut the power on a moment's notice, or there could be serious safety implications. To help ensure competent construction staff, an organization should work with its general contractor to provide comprehensive education and training. Some issues to cover within this training include the following:

- Life safety risks and ILSM
- Infection control risks and measures to address those risks
- Security issues
- Parking and building access
- Patient privacy
- Proper waste handling
- Cell phone use
- Equipment and materials
- Radiation safety, if applicable
- Hazardous materials
- Utility/electrical safety
- Smoking
- Violence prevention: How to seek help and report issues

surveyor. [9–10] "Yes," responds the facility manager. "The exit on the east side of the building is not useable, so we have posted signs throughout the area about alternative exits from the building. This helps us inform people who would normally use that exit how to navigate their way out of the building quickly in case of an emergency."

The facility manager goes on to talk about other ILSM the organization has in place around the construction site, including smoke-tight temporary construction partitions as well as increased surveillance of the area, which is maintained even during off-hours and on weekends. He mentions that the organization posts these measures on bulletin boards placed near the entrance to the construction site and on the organization's Web site. [11–12]

The surveyor then asks about fire drills involving the construction site. The facility manager discusses the most recent fire drill and describes how frequently the organization conducts such fire drills. [13–14]

The surveyor probes for further details on how the facility manager conducts routine rounds of the construction site: Who participates in those rounds? How long do they take? What is examined during the rounds? How frequently do they occur? The facility manager shows the surveyor a form he uses on the rounds to make sure he checks all the important aspects of the project and doesn't overlook anything. [15–20]

➜ *At the Construction Site.* After his conversation with the facility manager, the surveyor asks to go visit the construction site. Together, the surveyor and facility manager walk the site, checking to see if ILSM are in place and watching out for unnecessary clutter, debris, and anything else that could present a life safety risk for the project. The surveyor also checks that the doors to the construction project open in the correct direction and that there are a sufficient number of fire extinguishers.

➜ *At the Office of the General Contractor.* After touring the site, the surveyor stops by the office of the general contractor, where he asks more questions about life safety. During this conversation, he focuses on how the general contractor ensures that every construction worker understands the life safety risks present in the project and how to minimize those risks. He asks specifically about the education provided to the construction staff. He is checking to see if the general contractor's perspective on education and its importance mirrors that of the facility manager. [21–24]

"Could you describe the education and training you provide construction staff before and during the project?" asks the surveyor. "Sure," says the general contractor, pulling out a logbook. "Initially, we gave everyone working on the project an orientation. This was a group training session that I ran along with the facility manager. I documented—in this book here—everyone who participated in the training. That way, I can assure the organization that everyone received the proper education before coming on site. For new topics or those that need further emphasis, I provide some training during the weekly construction meeting. Sometimes the facility manager or the infection preventionist comes and talks during that meeting as well."

The surveyor follows up this answer with a few more questions about the project, ILSM, and fire drills. [25] On his way out of the general contractor's office, the surveyor stops a construction worker and asks him what education he's received about this project. Again, the surveyor is looking to see if everyone involved in the project understands the life safety risks present and how to minimize those risks. [26–27]

➜ *On a Patient Care Unit Near the Construction Site.* Finally, the surveyor stops by the patient care unit located nearest to the construction site. He speaks with a nurse manager there about the construction project, what impact it's had on the patient care unit, and whether the manager perceives increased life safety risks associated with the project. The surveyor asks about the signs showing alternative exits and whether debris, dust, and noise are problems in the area. The surveyor wants to know if the organization has considered and mitigated the impacts of the project on the patient care area nearby. [28–31]

MOCK TRACER TIP

As with many actual tracers, the key to conducting a mock tracer on life safety in a construction project is confirming that all members of the construction team—the general contractor, the construction workers, and the representative from the health care organization—are all on the same page regarding life safety risks, mitigation efforts, and the importance of education. It is not enough to interview the organization's liaison on a project; surveyors on mock tracers should also spend time talking with the general contractor and individuals working directly on the site.

➔ *Moving Forward.* Based on the tracer, the surveyor might follow up with a discussion about how and to whom the nurse manager reports any construction-related lapses in safety and how to stay alert for such lapses, report them appropriately, and follow up on what is being done to address them. [32–33]

Scenario 9-1.
Sample Tracer Questions

The bracketed numbers before each question correlate to questions, observations, and data review described in the sample tracer for Scenario 9-1. You can use the tracer worksheet form in Appendix B to develop a mock tracer (*see* an example of a completed tracer worksheet at the end of this section). The information gained by conducting a mock tracer can help to highlight a good practice and/or determine issues that may require further follow-up.

Facility Manager

[1] When did the project start? How long is it expected to continue?

[2] Has the organization experienced any problems in the project that could threaten the safety of patients, staff, and visitors? If so, describe them.

[3] Is there a "no smoking" policy for the area?

[4] How is that policy enforced?

[5] What training and orientation does the organization offer to construction workers?

[6] What topics are covered in that training?

[7] How is the training provided?

[8] How does the organization ensure that construction workers understand the training?

[9] Are any building exits compromised by the construction?

[10] What does the organization do to alert staff, visitors, and patients about alternate exits?

[11] What ILSM are present in the construction area?

[12] How does the organization notify patients, staff, and visitors about these ILSM?

[13] Does the organization do fire drills for this area?

[14] How often does the organization do them? When was the last one?

[15] How does the organization conduct rounds of the construction site?

[16] Who participates in these rounds?

[17] How long do the rounds take?

[18] What information are you looking for in these rounds?

[19] How frequently do the rounds occur?

[20] Do you document information observed in these rounds?

General Contractor

[21] How does the construction company preserve life safety on this site?

[22] How do you ensure that every construction worker understands the life safety risks present in the project and how to minimize those risks?

[23] What education do you provide to construction workers before and during the project?

[24] Do you document that education? If so, how?

[25] When was your most recent fire drill in this area? How did it go?

Construction Worker

[26] What education have you received about this project?

[27] Describe how you preserve life safety in this area.

Nurse Manager

[28] What impact has the construction project had on the patient care unit?

[29] Do you perceive increased life safety risks associated with the project?

[30] Are there signs showing alternate exits? Are patients and families ever confused when leaving the area?

[31] Are debris, dust, and noise problems in the area?

[32] How do you report a safety issue with the construction project?

[33] To whom would you report this issue?

SCENARIO 9-2. Interim Life Safety Measures (ILSM)

Summary

In the following scenario, a surveyor traces how an organization ensures the effective and appropriate use of ILSM to preserve life safety throughout the organization. Within the tracer, the surveyor explores issues relating to these priority focus areas:

- Communication
- Orientation and Training
- Patient Safety
- Physical Environment

Scenario

As a surveyor conducts a patient tracer, she notices that there is computer equipment installation going on nearby. She stops to observe the person performing the installation and notices that he inadvertently compromises a fire-rated barrier. Wanting to know how the organization's ILSM policy would govern its response to this situation, the surveyor decides to trace the issue.

(Bracketed numbers correlate to Sample Tracer Questions on pages 141–142.)

➜ *At the Office of the Facility Manager.* The surveyor begins her tracer at the office of the facility manager, where she asks him a series of questions about the organization's ILSM policy. Specifically, she wants to learn how the organization creates the policy, who's involved in creating it, who approves it, and whether it involves more than just life safety deficiencies associated with construction. She asks the facility manager to describe the situations in which the ILSM policy would go into effect. [1–5]

"Does this policy outline what measures are needed in certain situations?" asks the surveyor. "No, not really," says the facility manager. "The policy describes different ILSM options for preserving life safety but remains fairly broad regarding implementation. With that said, it does include written criteria for evaluating various deficiencies and construction hazards to determine when and to what extent the different ILSM apply. When there is a deficiency, either the safety officer or I will take a look at the deficiency and choose what activities will address and reduce the level of risk based on the policy. Usually, these activities don't apply to the whole building—just the area affected by the deficiency."

> ## MOCK TRACER TIP
>
> When conducting a mock tracer on how an organization uses ILSM to respond to a *Life Safety Code®** deficiency, it can be helpful to review any documentation associated with this implementation effort. Such documentation will show when and how an organization implemented and discontinued ILSM, and this can clearly illustrate compliance with the "Life Safety" (LS) chapter standards associated with this topic.

The surveyor follows up this answer by asking how the organization makes staff members, such as maintenance personnel, aware of the ILSM policy, how to access the policy, and what the policy contains. She also asks how the organization educates staff on reporting any life safety deficiencies. [6–7]

➜ *Reviewing the ILSM Policy.* The surveyor requests a copy of the ILSM policy. While reviewing it, she asks the facility manager to describe what would happen if someone discovered a *Life Safety Code* deficiency, such as the penetrated fire barrier she noticed earlier. How would the organization activate the policy? Who would make decisions about the appropriate measures? How would the organization document what measures it used? She also wants to determine how the organization enforces the policy, such as whether environment of care (EC) leaders conduct regular rounds of the ILSM to make sure they are in place and being used appropriately and consistently. In addition, she asks how the organization would know to stop using the measures once the deficiency is resolved. [8–13]

"Does the organization proactively look for *Life Safety Code* deficiencies?" asks the surveyor. [14] "Of course," says the facility manager. "We use the Statement of Conditions (SOC), environmental tours process, EC committee meeting minutes, and staff reports to identify potential deficiencies and respond to them. I also look pretty closely at any construction and renovation projects—no matter how small—that we may have under way."

Next, the surveyor asks some questions about how frequently the facility manager reviews these sources of information and what he does with the information gleaned from this review. [15–16]

Finally, the surveyor asks how the organization posts information about the particular ILSM used to mitigate a deficiency.

---

*Life Safety Code *is a registered trademark of the National Fire Protection Association, Quincy, MA.*

[17] The facility manager describes the posters the organization uses in patient care areas and staff break rooms. He adds that the organization includes information about any ILSM on its external and internal Web sites.

➡ *At an ILSM Location.* At the close of this conversation, the surveyor asks to go see an area where ILSM are currently in place. At this location, the surveyor reviews the ILSM. She notes the poster on the wall that explains them and how long the organization anticipates that they will be in place. While here, she chats with an individual working in the area to determine whether this person understands the ILSM and the reasons behind them. [18–21]

➡ *In the Maintenance Department.* As a final stop, the surveyor goes to the maintenance department and talks with one of the maintenance workers on duty. She asks him to describe a possible *Life Safety Code* deficiency that he may encounter. Specifically, she probes for details on how the maintenance worker would report the deficiency and use ILSM to respond to it. She wants to establish that the organization has a consistent approach to using ILSM and that staff members are aware of and familiar with this approach. [22–25]

➡ *Moving Forward.* Based on the tracer, the surveyor might follow up with a discussion about how organization staff—both maintenance personnel and frontline staff—could benefit from some further training and education around the topic of ILSM, specifically, when to use ILSM besides with a construction project.

At-a-glance
Compliance Strategies

Not every *Life Safety Code* deficiency warrants the same combination of ILSM. EC leaders, such as the safety officer or facility manager, must make decisions about what ILSM to implement in responding to a deficiency. As part of the decision-making process, leaders should work with staff members in the area where ILSM are needed because these individuals are often familiar with the location and the needs of the staff and patients within that location. They also may identify some obstacles in implementing ILSM that need to be addressed.

Scenario 9-2.
Sample Tracer Questions

The bracketed numbers before each question correlate to questions, observations, and data review described in the sample tracer for Scenario 9-2. You can use the tracer worksheet form in Appendix B to develop a mock tracer (*see* an example of a completed tracer worksheet at the end of this section). The information gained by conducting a mock tracer can help to highlight a good practice and/or determine issues that may require further follow-up.

Facility Manager

[1] How does the organization create its ILSM policy?

[2] Who is involved in creating this policy?

[3] Who approves this policy?

[4] Does the policy involve more than just life safety deficiencies associated with construction?

[5] Describe the situations in which the ILSM policy would go into effect.

[6] How does the organization make staff members, such as maintenance personnel, aware of the ILSM policy, how to access the policy, and what the policy contains?

[7] How does the organization educate staff on reporting any life safety deficiencies?

[8] Describe what would happen if someone discovered a *Life Safety Code* deficiency.

[9] How would the organization activate the ILSM policy?

[10] Who would make decisions about the appropriate measures?

[11] How would this decision maker document what measures were used?

[12] How does the organization enforce its ILSM policy?

[13] How would the organization know to stop using ILSM when a deficiency is resolved?

[14] Describe how the organization proactively looks for *Life Safety Code* deficiencies.

[15] How frequently do you review sources of information such as your SOC, environmental tours process, EC committee meeting minutes, and staff reports?

[16] What do you do with the information gleaned from this review?

(continued)

Scenario 9-2.
Sample Tracer Questions (continued)

[17] How does the organization post information about the particular ILSM used to mitigate a deficiency?

Unit Worker

[18] What are ILSM?

[19] What ILSM are in place in this unit?

[20] Why are they in place?

[21] How do they affect your daily routine?

Maintenance Worker

[22] Describe a possible *Life Safety Code* deficiency that you may encounter.

[23] How would you respond to that deficiency?

[24] How would you report the deficiency?

[25] How would you use ILSM to address the issue?

SCENARIO 9-3. Building Tours

Summary

In the following scenario, a surveyor conducts an organization's *Life Safety Code* building tour. Within the tracer, the surveyor explores issues relating to these priority focus areas:

• Communication
• Physical Environment

Scenario

During the on-site survey of a recently reconstructed health care organization, a *Life Safety Code* Specialist conducts a building tour to evaluate the effectiveness of the organization's processes for designing and maintaining buildings to *Life Safety Code* requirements.

(Bracketed numbers correlate to Sample Tracer Questions on pages 144–145.)

➡ *Reviewing the Documents.* Prior to conducting the tour, the surveyor reviews key documents related to life safety: the SOC, life safety drawings, fire-suppression system records, alarm-testing logs, fire drill records, and ILSM policies. He then meets with several EC leaders in the organization, including the

facility manager—who is in charge of fire safety—and the safety officer. He asks them to describe the organization's approach to life safety, including how the organization ensures compartmentalization. [1]

After this discussion, the group visits different areas of the organization, where the surveyor looks to see how the facility complies with *Life Safety Code* requirements. During this time, the surveyor also asks the EC leaders some questions about *Life Safety Code* compliance efforts.

➡ *Within Hazardous Areas.* The surveyor first visits several hazardous areas, including soiled linen rooms, trash collection rooms, and oxygen storage rooms. While in these locations, he asks about the fire ratings of the perimeter walls and doors in these areas as well as about the latching and closing abilities of the doors. He makes sure that any storage rooms larger than 100 square feet have perimeter walls that are one-hour fire rated and doors that self-close and latch. [2–3]

➡ *Examining Fire Walls and Doors.* Next, the surveyor walks through other areas of the facility, looking at fire walls and doors. He checks to see if building separations have a two-hour fire rating and extend from the floor slab to the floor or roof slab above and from the outside edge of the building to the opposing outside edge. He stops to look at several fire wall doors and asks the EC leaders what the fire ratings are for the doors. He also checks whether the doors swing in the correct direction—toward the path of egress. [4–6]

"Could you describe how these fire doors close?" asks the surveyor. [7] "All our fire doors close and latch and have self-closing or automatic-closing capability, meaning that when someone or something passes through a door opening, the door automatically closes and latches," says the facility manager. "For some of our doors, we use an electromagnetic device that ties into our alarm system. When the alarm sounds, the electromagnetic device disengages, and the doors automatically close and latch."

The surveyor follows up this answer by asking about the gap allowed between fire doors as well as the gap between the bottom edge of the doors and the floor. He also asks about protective plates—both their purpose and their appropriate size and material. [8–9]

As the surveyor walks through the building, he notices that several patient room doors have holiday decorations hanging from them. He points out that these are not allowed per the

Life Safety (LS) standards because any doors that are fire rated at ¾ hour or longer must be kept free from decorations, coverings, and other objects. [10]

Finally, the surveyor examines some penetrations in the fire-rated walls involving pipes, conduits, cables, and wires. He asks what fire-rated material the organization uses as a fire stop and whether that material has been approved by a designated testing agency, such as Underwriters Laboratories (UL). [11–12]

➡ *Examining Smoke Compartments.* Next, the surveyor looks at smoke compartments and verifies that there are at least two such compartments for every story in the building that has patient sleeping or treatment rooms. He asks about the doors in smoke barriers and whether they are self-closing or automatic closing. He presses for information about spaces between the smoke doors and the appropriate size of protective plates used on these doors. [13–14]

➡ *Looking at Corridors.* As the surveyor is touring the building, he makes note of the exit corridors, verifying that they are at least 8 feet wide. He looks at both the corridor walls and doors, checking to see that they are constructed in the appropriate sizes and materials. During this time, the surveyor asks how the organization keeps its corridors free from clutter, such as stored furniture, construction material, and equipment that is not in use. He notices that there is a housekeeping cart in one of the hallways. [15–18]

"Do you normally store housekeeping carts in the hallway?" asks the surveyor. "Only when the cart is in use," says the safety officer. "That means we can only store it there if it is used every 30 minutes. So, when the housekeeping staff members are actively cleaning rooms, we allow them to store the carts there. Otherwise, the carts need to be stored off the exit corridor."

The surveyor then asks about other carts, such as crash carts, and whether they are stored in the hallway.

➡ *Looking at the Automatic Sprinkler System.* The surveyor then examines the automatic sprinkler equipment in the building to make sure there is appropriate space under sprinkler heads. He also verifies that the sprinkler system piping is safe, secure, and free of damage. He notes that some of the piping is not as securely attached to the ceiling as it should be and mentions this to the facility manager. He suggests reviewing the security of the piping during environmental tours

to identify piping that needs to be more secure. He comments that proactively addressing this issue can prevent the piping from dislodging or breaking apart when the sprinklers engage. [19–20]

➡ *At the Exit Stairs.* Next, the surveyor asks to see the exit stairs, where he verifies that the stairs are continuous from the highest level they serve to the outside of the building. While doing this, he asks about the fire rating for the exit stairs. He also tries to determine how the organization ensures proper signage in the area. He then verifies that the stairwell exit discharges to a safe location and asks the organization how it maintains egress through the passageway to a public way. [21–25]

➡ *At the Kitchen.* The surveyor visits the kitchen and looks at how the organization addresses life safety there. He examines the fire-suppression system in the exhaust hood. He also checks to see that there are portable K-type fire extinguishers—a specific type of extinguisher designed to suppress grease

At-a-glance
Compliance Strategies

A key concept in designing and maintaining a building to comply with the *Life Safety Code* is compartmentalization. This is the idea that organizations must use various building components—fire-rated walls and doors, smoke barriers, fire-rated floor slabs—to prevent the spread of fire and the products of combustion. By compartmentalizing a building, an organization can restrict the movement of fire from one part of the building to another, provided that adequate barriers are maintained. This allows for a "defend-in-place" fire strategy, in which the building and fire-suppression systems protect the occupants for a predetermined amount of time. If evacuation is necessary, the compartmentalization ensures safe passage out of one compartment to another or out of the building.

When examining compliance efforts with regard to the *Life Safety Code*, an organization should take an overall view of compartmentalization to make sure all components of the building are working together to prevent the spread of fire.

fires—within 30 feet of the exhaust hood equipment. The surveyor then asks whether the automatic sprinklers in this area are linked to the master fire alarm panel as well as whether fuel sources automatically shut off in the event of a fire. He probes for details about how the exhaust/duct system functions in this area, trying to assess whether the system functions as it was designed to function. **[26–30]**

➡ *In a Laundry Room.* Next, the surveyor stops by one of the organization's laundry areas and asks about the laundry chute: How does the sprinkler system in the chute work? How do the doors to the chute and the doors to the room housing the chute work? What are the fire ratings of the chute walls and the discharge door from the laundry chute? Is the laundry area used for other purposes besides laundry? **[31–34]**

➡ *At the Master Fire Alarm Panel.* The next stop is the master alarm panel in the organization's lobby, where the surveyor asks a few more questions. "Is this area continually monitored?" asks the surveyor.

"No, but we do have a smoke detector placed very near the alarm panel that would alert us in case of a problem," says the facility manager. "We also have a secondary panel that is safe, protected, and located near the organization switchboard. This helps us ensure that the fire alarm monitoring system will still function even if there is a fire in the location of the master alarm panel." **[35–36]**

The surveyor asks why the organization chose these locations for its alarm panels and whether the panels have ever been moved. He then asks how the organization transmits a fire alarm notification to the local authorities. **[37–39]**

➡ *At the Power Plant.* Finally, the surveyor assesses the condition of the organization's emergency power systems and equipment. He verifies that there is a reliable emergency power system that supplies electricity to exit signs, emergency/urgent care areas, areas with life support equipment, operating rooms, and similar vital systems. **[40]**

Before ending the tour, the surveyor takes note of the paths of egress throughout the facility, making sure that exit hallways, signs, stairways, doors, and discharge areas are adequately lit. **[41]**

➡ *Moving Forward.* At the close of the tour, the surveyor reviews his notes from the tour and conducts a verbal interview with the EC leaders about areas of success and areas that need improvement.

MOCK TRACER TIP

Most of the standards in the LS chapter of the Joint Commission's Comprehensive Accreditation Manuals are designed to mirror the requirements of the *Life Safety Code* and are laid out by occupancy type. When conducting a mock building tour, it can be helpful to use the LS standards to guide the content of the tour and the questions to ask within the tour.

The Joint Commission does not require freestanding business occupancies to comply with the *Life Safety Code*. However, such facilities must still maintain free and unobstructed access to all exits. When conducting a mock tracer on life safety in these occupancies, an organization can focus on how it maintains access to exits and conducts regular fire drills.

Scenario 9-3.
Sample Tracer Questions

The bracketed numbers before each question correlate to questions, observations, and data review described in the sample tracer for Scenario 9-3. You can use the tracer worksheet form in Appendix B to develop a mock tracer (*see* an example of a completed tracer worksheet at the end of this section). The information gained by conducting a mock tracer can help to highlight a good practice and/or determine issues that may require further follow-up.

EC Leaders

[1]   Describe the organization's approach to life safety, including how it ensures compartmentalization.

[2]   What are the fire ratings of the perimeter walls and doors in hazardous areas?

[3]   What are the latching and closing abilities of doors in these areas?

[4]   Do building separations have a two-hour fire rating and extend from the floor slab to the floor or roof slab above and from the outside edge of the building to the opposing outside edge?

[5]   What is the fire rating for fire wall doors?

[6] Do fire wall doors swing in the correct direction?

[7] Describe how fire wall doors close.

[8] What gap is allowed between fire doors? between the bottom edge of the doors and the floor?

[9] Describe the purpose, size, and material of protective plates used on fire doors.

[10] Are patient room doors (and other doors) kept free from decorations, coverings, and other objects?

[11] What fire-rated material does the organization use as a fire stop?

[12] Has that material been approved by a designated testing agency, such as UL?

[13] Are there two smoke compartments for every story with patient sleeping or treatment rooms?

[14] Describe the doors in smoke barriers, including their ability to close, spacing, material, and protective plates.

[15] What is the width between walls in exit corridors?

[16] Describe the doors in exit corridors.

[17] How does the organization keep its corridors free from clutter?

[18] What types of carts can be stored in exit corridors?

[19] Is there appropriate space under all sprinkler heads?

[20] Is all sprinkler system piping safe, secure, and free of damage?

[21] Are exit stairs continuous from the highest level they serve to the outside of the building?

[22] What is the fire rating for exit stairs?

[23] How does the organization ensure proper signage in exit stairs?

[24] Does the stairwell exit discharge to a safe location?

[25] How does the organization maintain the exit through the passageway to a public way?

[26] How does the organization maintain life safety in the kitchen?

[27] Are there portable K-type fire extinguishers within 30 feet of the exhaust hood equipment?

[28] Are the automatic sprinklers in this area linked to the master fire alarm panel?

[29] Would fuel sources automatically shut off in the event of a fire?

[30] Describe how the exhaust/duct system functions in this area.

[31] Describe the sprinkler system in the laundry chute.

[32] How do the doors to the chute and the doors to the room housing the chute work?

[33] What are the fire ratings of the chute walls and the discharge door from the laundry chute?

[34] Is the laundry area used for other purposes besides laundry?

[35] Is the area around the master fire alarm panel continually monitored, or is there a smoke detector in the area?

[36] Where is the secondary alarm panel located?

[37] Why did the organization choose these locations?

[38] Have the panels ever been moved?

[39] How does the organization transmit a fire alarm notification to the local authorities?

[40] Is there a reliable emergency power system that supplies electricity to exit signs, emergency/urgent care areas, areas with life support equipment, operating rooms, and so on?

[41] Are paths of egress adequately lit?

Sample Tracer Worksheet: Scenario 9-2.

The worksheet below is an example of how organizations can use the sample tracer questions for Scenario 9-2 in a worksheet format during a mock tracer. The bracketed numbers before each question correlate to questions described in the scenario.

A **correct answer** is an appropriate answer that meets the requirements of the organization and other governing bodies. An **incorrect answer** should always include recommendations for follow-up.

Tracer Team Member(s): Catherine Parker
Subjects Interviewed: Thomas Beebe, Doris Brown, Max Chang
Tracer Topic: ILSM

Data Record(s): logs of actual implementation of ILSM
Unit(s) or Department(s): Facility manager's office, ILSM location on 8W, maintenance department

Interview Subject: Facility Manager

Questions	Correct Answer	Incorrect Answer	Follow-Up Needed	Comments or Notes
[1–4] How does the organization create its ILSM policy? Who is involved in creating it? Who approves it? Does the policy involve more than just life safety deficiencies associated with construction?	✓			Organization uses Joint Commission standards to help design the policy. Involves both EC professionals and leadership in creating the policy. Board approves the policy. Does address more than just construction.
[5] Describe the situations in which the ILSM policy would go into effect.		✓	Could use some further training on when the ILSM policy should go into effect.	Able to describe some scenarios well. I pointed out others with which he was not familiar.
[6–7] How does the organization make staff members, such as maintenance personnel, aware of the ILSM policy, how to access the policy, and what the policy contains?		✓	As mentioned before, need to work on training personnel on ILSM policy.	Don't have formal processes for educating people in the organization on the ILSM policy.

Interview Subject: *Facility Manager (continued)*				
Question	**Correct Answer**	**Incorrect Answer**	**Follow-Up Needed**	**Comments or Notes**
[8–11] Describe what would happen if someone discovered a *Life Safety Code* deficiency. How would the organization activate the ILSM policy? Who would make decisions about the appropriate measures? How would this decision maker document what measures were used?	✓			Able to describe how the policy would be activated, who would make the decision about appropriate ILSM, and how the ILSM would be documented.
[13] How would the organization know to stop using ILSM when a deficiency is resolved?		✓	Consider defining a process to ensure that ILSM are stopped when no longer necessary.	Doesn't have a good way of keeping track of this. If the facility manager notices during rounds that ILSM should be stopped, he stops them. Otherwise, they could go on longer than they should.
[14–16] Describe how the organization proactively looks for *Life Safety Code* deficiencies. How frequently do you review sources of information such as your SOC, environmental tours process, EC committee meeting minutes, and staff reports? What do you do with information gleaned from this review?		✓	Should consider developing a more formal ILSM risk assessment that includes a multidisciplinary approach and occurs on a more regular basis. Part of this assessment could focus on responding to risks identified.	Although the facility manager uses the SOC, EC committee minutes, environmental tours, and staff reporting, the process is a little haphazard. Facility manager cannot say how often he reviews this information, and there is no formal process for responding to the information.
[17] How does the organization post information about the particular ILSM used to mitigate a deficiency?	✓			The organization does a nice job with posters and information on the internal and external Web sites.

(continued)

Interview Subject: Unit Worker				
Questions	**Correct Answer**	**Incorrect Answer**	**Follow-Up Needed**	**Comments or Notes**
[18–21] Describe what ILSM are, what specific ILSM are in place on this unit, why they are in place, and how they affect your job.		✓	Work on improving communication with staff about ILSM and why ILSM are important. Acknowledge that ILSM can be inconvenient sometimes but are necessary to preserve patient and staff safety.	Staff member cannot adequately describe what ILSM are. She knows there are some things different on the unit that relate to fire prevention but can't articulate the specifics. She does mention that it's been complicated getting around the area, and the new things in the unit have made her job more difficult.

Interview Subject: Maintenance Worker				
Questions	**Correct Answer**	**Incorrect Answer**	**Follow-Up Needed**	**Comments or Notes**
[22, 23, 25] Describe a possible *Life Safety Code* deficiency that you may encounter. How would you respond to that deficiency? How would you use ILSM to address the issue?	✓			Maintenance staff seem more familiar than frontline staff with the concept of ILSM and how to address *Life Safety Code* deficiencies using ILSM.
[24] How would you report a *Life Safety Code* deficiency?	✓			Can describe a well-considered reporting process. Should share this process with other staff in the organization.

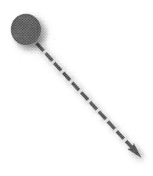

Appendix A   Priority Focus Areas

Priority Focus Areas

At the beginning of each tracer scenario in this workbook is a brief summary that includes the priority focus areas (PFAs) that are focused on in the scenario. The PFAs are processes, systems, or structures in a health care organization that significantly impact safety and/or the quality of care provided. There are 14 PFAs that are generally universal across health care settings. All Joint Commission standards are related to PFAs. During the onsite survey process, surveyors link the PFAs within standards compliance issues to identify potential areas of risk. The PFAs, along with clinical/service groups (CSGs) from the Priority Focus Process (PFP), form the foundation of the tracer process. The CSGs categorize care recipients and/or services into distinct populations for which data can be collected. The PFP is a data-driven tool that helps focus survey activity on issues most relevant to care recipient safety and quality of care at the specific health care organization being surveyed.

The PFAs related to environment of care are summarized in the following sections.

Assessment & Care/Services

Assessment & Care/Services for care recipients comprise the execution of a series of processes that are fluid in nature to accommodate needs of care recipients including, as relevant, screening; assessment; planning care, treatment, and/or services; provision of care; ongoing reassessment of care; and discharge planning, referral for continuing care, or discontinuation of services. Although some elements of Assessment & Care/Services may occur only once, other aspects may be repeated or revisited as the care recipient's needs or care delivery priorities change. Successful implementation of improvements in Assessment & Care/Services relies on the full support of leadership.

Subprocesses of Assessment & Care/Services include the following:
- Screening

- Assessment
- Planning care, treatment, or services
- Provision of care, treatment, or services
- Reassessment
- Discharge planning or discontinuation of services

Communication

Communication is the process by which information is exchanged between individuals, programs/services, or organizations. Effective Communication successfully permeates every aspect of a health care organization, from the provision of care to performance improvement, resulting in a marked improvement in the quality of care delivery and functioning.

Subprocesses of Communication include the following:
- Provider and/or staff–care recipient communication
- Care recipient and family education
- Staff communication and collaboration
- Information dissemination
- Multidisciplinary teamwork

Credentialed Practitioners

Credentialed Practitioners are health care professionals whose qualifications to provide care, treatment, and services have been verified and assessed, resulting in the assignment of clinical responsibilities. The Credentialed Practitioners category varies from organization to organization and from state to state. It includes licensed independent practitioners and others who are permitted to provide care, treatment, and services to care recipients under the direction of a sponsoring physician. Licensed independent practitioners are permitted by law and the health care organization to provide care, treatment, and services without clinical supervision or direction within the scope of their license and consistent with individually assigned clinical responsibilities or individually granted privileges.

Equipment Use

Equipment Use incorporates the selection, delivery, setup, and maintenance of equipment and supplies to meet the needs of care recipients and staff. It generally includes movable equipment, as well as management of supplies that staff members use (for example, gloves, syringes). (Equipment Use does not include fixed equipment such as built-in oxygen and gas lines and central air conditioning systems; such items are included in the Physical Environment PFA.) Equipment Use includes planning and selecting; training and orientation; maintaining, testing, and inspecting; educating and providing instructions; delivery and setup; and risk prevention related to equipment and/or supplies. NOTE: This PFA is not applicable to Behavioral Health Care accreditation programs.

Subprocesses of Equipment Use include the following:
- Selection
- Maintenance strategies
- Periodic evaluation
- Orientation and training

Infection Control

Infection Control includes the prevention, surveillance/identification, and control of infections among care recipients, employees, physicians and other licensed independent practitioners, contract service workers, volunteers, students, and visitors. Infection Control is a systemwide, integrated process that is applied to all programs, services, and settings.

Subprocesses of Infection Control include the following:
- Prevention and control
- Surveillance/identification
- Reporting
- Measurement

Orientation & Training

Orientation is the process of educating newly hired staff in health care organizations to organizationwide, department, program-, service-, and jobspecific competencies before they provide care, treatment, or services to care recipients. Newly hired staff includes, but is not limited to, regular staff employees, contracted staff, agency (temporary) staff, float staff, volunteer staff, students, housekeeping, and maintenance staff.

Training refers to the development and implementation of programs that foster staff development and continued learning, address skill deficiencies, and thereby help ensure staff retention. More specifically, training entails providing opportunities for staff to develop enhanced skills related to revised processes that may have been addressed during orientation, new care techniques for care recipients, or expanded job responsibilities. Whereas orientation is a one-time process, training is a continuous one.

Subprocesses of Orientation & Training include the following:
- Organizationwide orientation
- Program/service orientation
- Job-specific orientation
- Training and continuing or ongoing education

Patient Safety

Patient Safety entails a framework for proactively identifying the potential and actual risks to safety, identifying the underlying cause(s) of the potential or actual risk, and making the necessary improvements to reduce risk. It also entails establishing processes to respond to sentinel events, identifying risks through root cause analysis, and making necessary improvements. This involves a systems-based approach that examines all activities within an organization that contribute to maintaining and improving care recipient safety, including performance improvement and risk management, to ensure that the activities work together, not independently, to improve care and safety. This systems-based approach is driven by organization leadership; anchored in the organization's mission, vision, and strategic plan; endorsed and actively supported by medical staff and nursing leadership; implemented by directors; integrated and coordinated throughout the organization's staff; and continuously re-engineered using proven, proactive performance improvement modalities. In addition, effective reduction of errors and other factors that contribute to unintended adverse outcomes in an organization requires an environment in which care recipients, their families, and organization staff and leaders can identify and manage actual and potential risks to safety.

Subprocesses of Patient Safety include the following:
- Planning and designing services
- Directing services
- Integrating and coordinating services
- Reducing and preventing errors
- Using Sentinel Event Alerts
- The Joint Commission National Patient Safety Goals
- Clinical practice guidelines, if available
- Actively involving care recipients in their care, treatment, or services

Physical Environment

The Physical Environment refers to a safe, accessible, functional, supportive, and effective physical environment for care recipients, staff members, workers, and others by managing physical design;

construction and redesign; maintenance and testing; planning and improvement; and risk prevention, defined in terms of utilities, fire protection, security, privacy, storage, and hazardous materials and waste. The Physical Environment may include the home in the case of in-home programs and foster care.

Subprocesses of Physical Environment include the following:
- Physical design
- Construction and redesign
- Maintenance and testing
- Planning and improvement
- Risk prevention

Quality Improvement Expertise/Activities

Quality Improvement Expertise/Activities identifies the collaborative and interdisciplinary approach to the continuous study and improvement of the processes of providing health care services to meet the needs of consumers and others. Quality Improvement Expertise depends on understanding and revising processes on the basis of data and knowledge about the processes themselves. Quality Improvement involves identifying, measuring, implementing, monitoring, analyzing, planning, and maintaining processes to ensure they function effectively. Examples of Quality Improvement Activities include designing a new service, flowcharting a clinical process, collecting and analyzing data about performance measures or care recipient outcomes, comparing the organization's performance to that of other organizations, selecting areas for priority attention, and experimenting with new ways of carrying out a function.

Subprocesses of Quality Improvement Expertise/Activities include the following:
- Identifying issues and establishing priorities
- Developing measures
- Collecting data to evaluate status on outcomes, processes, or structures
- Analyzing and interpreting data
- Making and implementing recommendations
- Monitoring and sustaining performance improvement

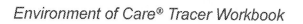

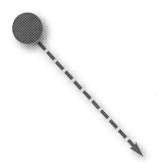

Appendix B Mock Tracer Worksheet Form

You can use the worksheet on the following pages to record information during a mock tracer. Make as many extra copies of the second page as needed. Below are explanations of terms on the worksheet.

Worksheet Terms

- **Mock Tracer Name:** Give your mock tracer a name for easy reference. This may be as simple as Mock Tracer 1.

- **Date(s) Conducted:** Indicate the date(s) on which the mock tracer took place.

- **Tracer Team Member(s):** List the person or people performing the tracers in the surveyor role.

- **Subjects Interviewed:** List all the people who were interviewed during the entire tracer.

- **Tracer Topic:** Note the topic traced by the person or people performing the surveyor role in the mock tracer. You may also think of it as the focus of the mock tracer.

- **Data Record(s):** List any documents—paper or electronic—consulted during the mock tracer.

- **Unit(s) or Department(s):** List all places visited during the mock tracer. They should conform to the places where the interview subjects work or were encountered during the tracer.

- **Interview Subject:** Fill in the name of the person interviewed. If the person is a member of the staff or administration, add his or her job title as well.

- **Questions:** Record each question asked of the particular interview subject. You might want to use some of the sample tracer questions from the scenarios in this workbook for mock tracers with a similar focus to those scenarios.

- **Correct Answer and Incorrect Answer:** Check the appropriate column to indicate whether the interview subject provided a correct or incorrect answer. A **correct answer** is an appropriate answer that meets the requirements of the organization and other governing bodies. An **incorrect answer** should always include recommendations for follow-up.

- **Follow-Up Needed:** When the interview subject gives an incorrect answer, specify follow-up. This may be recommendations for further evaluation of an issue, staff education, or even another mock tracer.

- **Comments or Notes:** Add anything else you need to remark on. Use this spot as a place to record positive impressions for correct answers as well.

Mock Tracer Name:
Date(s) Conducted:
Tracer Team Member(s):

Subjects Interviewed:

Tracer Topic:
Data Record(s):

Unit(s) or Department(s):

Interview Subject:

Questions	Correct Answer	Incorrect Answer	Follow-Up Needed	Comments or Notes

Interview Subject:				
Questions	**Correct Answer**	**Incorrect Answer**	**Follow-Up Needed**	**Comments or Notes**

Interview Subject:				
Questions	**Correct Answer**	**Incorrect Answer**	**Follow-Up Needed**	**Comments or Notes**

Index